COMMUNICATION
APPREHENSION
ORIGINS AND MANAGEMENT

Stephanie S. Eley

DEDICATION

To my most valuable teachers of all—the students and patients
who inspired this book

COMMUNICATION APPREHENSION
ORIGINS AND MANAGEMENT

Betty Horwitz, Ed.D.
Private Practice
New York, New York

SINGULAR

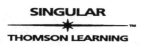

THOMSON LEARNING

Australia Canada Mexico Singapore Spain United Kingdom United States

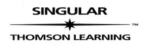

SINGULAR

TM

THOMSON LEARNING

Communication Apprehension: Origins and Management

Betty Horwitz, Ed.D.

Business Unit Director: William Brotmiller	**Editorial Assistant:** Cara Jenkins	**Production Coordinator:** John Mickelbank
Acquisitions Editor: Marie Linvill	**Project Editor:** Mary Ellen Cox	**Art/Design Coordinator:** Timothy J. Conners

Library of Congress Cataloging-in-Publication Data

Horwitz, Betty.
Communication apprehension: origins and management/Betty Horwitz.
p.cm.
Includes bibliographical references and index.
ISBN 1-56593-924-7
(alk. paper)
1. Performance anxiety.
2. Fear. 3. Stress (Psychology) 4. Stress management. I. Title.\
BF575.A6 H675 2001
616.85'22--dc21

2001017479

NOTICE TO READER

CONTENTS

PREFACE

There has been a plethora of books on communication disorders but few offer substantive information on how anxiety affects the ability to communicate or the relationship between thoughts, feelings, physiological responses and speaking. It is hoped that this book will fill that gap, in part, by exploring that interconnection and the resulting communication apprehension, a serious clinical concern that epitomizes the mind-body connection.

The primary purpose of the book is to demystify the devastating fear of performance suffered by millions of people and to help them cope with the problem. It addresses the origins and management of what is known in the psychiatric world as a social phobia, a common type of anxiety disorder that is generally hidden and neglected.

The book is written primarily for speech-language pathologists who will learn about the mind-body connection and its importance in the assessment of communication apprehension as well as other communication disorders. However, it will also benefit educators, performing artist mentors and corporate trainers who should be able to adapt the information on performance anxiety reduction for their populations. The book examines communication apprehension from several perspectives: developmental, psychological physiological and management.

Chapter 1 introduces the topic of communication apprehension by describing the reactions, problems and demographics of this universal fear. This is followed by an overview of anxiety and anxiety disorders leading to an explanation of social phobia (communication apprehension/performance anxiety), the fear of evaluation by others. This problem is considered to be a hidden communication disorder.

Examples of persons with communication disorders and so-called "normal" speakers who suffer communication apprehension are presented. The chapter includes professional concerns and a rationale for voice and speech-language clinicians to become involved with the problem.

Chapter 2 addresses the developmental perspectives of communication apprehension by answering several pertinent questions related to its etiology. It begins by considering the role of brain wiring and evolution in the fear response and addresses the reasons for social fears. It then discusses individual differences and the cognitive/behavioral role in the emergence of communication apprehension. This is followed by a discussion of the influence of culture and other factors related to the emergence of this common fear.

Chapter 3, the psychological perspective, is an in-depth discussion of the identification of and intervention in anxiety and anxiety disorders for speech pathologists by Dr. Donald Moss, eminent psychologist and president-elect of the Association of Applied Psychophysiology and Biofeedback (AAPB). Beginning with information on the diagnosis of anxiety, it summarizes the classifications of anxiety disorders and provides a screening procedure for them. This is followed by a comprehensive overview of therapeutic interventions for anxiety disorders and an elaboration of the problem of social phobia introduced in Chapter 1.

Chapter 4 presents the physiological perspective of stress, which explains the symptoms of communication apprehension. Dr. Richard Gevirtz, professor at the California School of Professional Psychology and leading researcher in psychophysiology, begins this chapter with an explanation of the transactional model of stress and recent views of the autonomic nervous system, which clarifies the intense reactions to social evaluation by humans. The roles of the endocrine and respiratory systems in the stress response are then discussed followed by the consequences of its prolonged activation. The chapter concludes with treatment implications for stress, which validates the physiological and cognitive/behavioral strategies used for the reduction of communication apprehension presented in this book.

Chapter 5 presents the management perspective for communication apprehension. It describes one university-affiliated program successfully used with adults whose fear primarily involved speaking in public. Its format, goals and targets, and agenda are presented, including a discussion of the communication environment, the role of the leader, and a detailed description of an 8-week class to overcome the fear of speaking. It is believed that this course can serve as a prototype for communication apprehension workshops with populations such as professional performers, school children, and corporate personnel. The last portion of the chapter discusses management techniques for communication apprehension. This is followed by recent advances in its treatment, including resonant frequency training, (respiratory/cardiovascular approach), and virtual reality.

The Epilogue briefly reviews some basic tenets related to understanding communication apprehension and reiterates the rationale for clinicians and the field of speech-language pathology at large to become involved in the problem.

I am indebted to many self-actualized people who guided me in this undertaking. I am especially grateful to Drs. Don Moss and Dick Gevirtz, two contributing authors, both psychologists par excellence, whose help has been invaluable and from whom I have learned so much. A special thanks to Dr. Ian Wickramasekera, an outstanding clinician and researcher, who has been an inspiration and mentor and to Dr. Alexander Smetankin of Biosyvaz, who opened up new vistas to me with his innovative physiological approach to anxiety reduction. Thanks also to Dr. Siggie and Sue Ottheimer of EEG Spectrum with whom I first learned about the power and ability to alter brain function with neural (brain wave) feedback and to Barbara Peavy, who guided me to the Association of Applied Psychophysiology and Biofeedback and whetted my appetite for more with her excellent workshop in stress management way back when.

I am also indebted to Dr. Sadanand Singh of Singular Publishing, who encouraged me to do something with my interests and to his excellent staff, Candice Janco and Marie Linvill. I also thank Pam Rider, my wonderful editor who kept me laughing while leading me gently through a maze of convoluted sentences and unending detail.

Thanks also to Robbie Paden, who critiqued the early manuscript versions and rescued me from countless computer fiascos while she ran my office and to Dr. Kay Monkhouse, Shirley Tennyson, and Flora Viale for their encouraging comments and feedback. I am also deeply grateful to my dear friend, Dr. Jim Perryman, (posthumous), for his steadfast belief in me and support of this endeavor. And last, but far from least, my gratitude goes to all of my students and patients throughout the years, who taught me so much, thereby enriching my life.

This has been a long and arduous journey but not without its rewards. Simply put, I see, hear, and feel differently. As a result, I believe that I am a more understanding person and effective clinician. I sincerely hope that the reader finds the topic of communication apprehension and its related topics as challenging, meaningful, and illuminating as I have.

B. Horwitz, Ed.D.

CONTRIBUTORS

Richard Gevirtz, Ph.D.
Professor of Health Psychology
California School of Professional Psychology at Alliant University
San Diego, California

Donald Moss, Ph.D.
Partner
West Michigan Behavioral Health Services
Grand Haven, Michigan

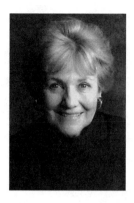

Communication Apprehension: Origins and Management

Betty Horwitz, Ed.D., CCC-SPL

About the Author

Dr. Betty Horwitz, a licensed speech pathologist in private practice in New York City, has been an adjunct professor for the past ten years at New York University where she received an award for teaching excellence. She received a B.A. (Speech Pathology) from the University of Michigan, an M.A. (Speech Pathology) from Kean University in New Jersey, and an M.A. (Developmental Psychology) and Ed.D. (Speech Pathology) from Columbia University. In addition, she had postdoctoral training in child and adolescent psychotherapy at the New Hope Guild in New York and in psychophysiology and biofeedback with the Association for Applied Psychophysiology and Biofeedback (AAPB). She is a certified stress management educator (BCIA), a contributor to the ASHA Prevention Manual, and among the inaugural cadre of fluency specialists with ASHA.

Dr. Horwitz has worked in rehabilitation centers, schools and clinics with varied speech, language and voice disorders and has been on the faculty of the Communication Disorders Departments of City College of New York, Southern Connecticut State University and more recently, Touro College in Brooklyn. She also has been a consultant and trainer in the private sector and with the Federal Emergency Management Agency for whom she developed a widely used program and textbook on Leadership and Oral Communication. Her experience and special interests in human development, stuttering and voice led Dr. Horwitz to explore the effects of anxiety on oral communications which she has written about and lectured on in the USA and abroad.

CHAPTER

1

Introduction and Overview: The Hidden Communication Problem

"But that isn't right. The King of Beasts shouldn't be a coward," said the Scarecrow.

"I know it," returned the Lion, wiping a tear from his eye with the tip of his tail. "It is my great sorrow, and makes my life very unhappy. But whenever there is danger, my heart begins to beat fast."

"Perhaps you have a heart disease," said the Woodsman.

"It may be," said the Lion.

L. Frank Baum, *The Wonderful Wizard of Oz*[1]

Communication apprehension, also known as stage fright, communication anxiety, or performance anxiety can easily be classified as "the hidden communication disorder," because it frequently is not recognized, acknowledged, or discussed. Communication apprehension is defined as anxiety or fear suffered by an individual of either actual or anticipated communication, with a group or a person, that can profoundly affect their oral communication, social skills, and self-esteem (Holbrook, 1987).

[1]From *The Wonderful Wizard of Oz* (p. 69), by L. F. Baum, 1987, New York: William Morrow and Company.

1

The treatment of communication apprehension is a natural fit for speech-language pathologists (SLPs), because many patients with clearly diagnosed communication disorders have anxiety about communicating that may or may not be related to their presenting problems. In addition, speaking anxiety is a common universal problem among people without communication disorders. For these reasons alone, the study of communication apprehension warrants the attention of speech-language pathologists who can, with additional training, easily develop the expertise to treat the multitude of people who suffer from this problem.

Some might argue that it is not within the domain of speech-language pathologists to include anxiety treatment in their therapeutic regimes because they are not mental health practitioners, per se. However, effective speech-language clinicians do not treat communication disorders, but rather persons with communication disorders. This approach necessitates understanding and incorporating the attitudes, beliefs, and feelings—the personal constructs—of people into the assessment and therapy of all patients. Moreover, many communication disorders are listed in the *Diagnostic and Statistical Manual of Mental Disorders (DSM-IV;* American Psychiatric Association, 1994). The list includes stuttering, pervasive developmental disorders, elective mutism, attention deficits, and dysphonia. Most significantly, speech-language pathologists already are concerned with mental health as they always work toward improving the self confidence of all patients while facilitating mastery of their communication skills. In so doing, they inevitably deal with issues of anxiety, an integral part of their clinical work.

However, even some well-established speech pathologists and vocologists do not understand or adequately manage the psychological and physiological effects of anxiety on their patients. This may be because their training has not included work in the ancient and modern concepts of the mind-body connection and the role of self-regulation in restoring mental and physical balance. This omission may be attributed, in part, to lack of awareness of advances in psychophysiology and behavioral medicine, to issues of professional territoriality, or to the assumption that SLPs work with mental health professionals in multidisciplinary settings.

There is no doubt that the most effective way to work with communication disorders is in a multidisciplinary setting with easy access to psychologists and social workers for consultation and collaboration. However, many speech language pathologists do not work in teams and health care systems often do not provide adequate referrals to mental health professionals, even if patients accept such recommendations. These are additional reasons why the study of anxiety in general, and communication apprehension in particular, is important for speech-language pathologists. Both clinicians and clients who suffer from these problems stand to gain from this broader professional horizon.

According to Marshall (1944), 30% to 40% of the general population considered public speaking their number one fear, surpassing fears of heights, sickness, loneliness, and the dark. This finding is corroborated by others who report that public speaking is the single most common fear regardless of age, sex, education level, or even preparation and social skills (Buss, 1980; Edelman, 1992; Roy-Byrne and Keaton, 1944; Slipman, 1986). Schneier (1993) reported that 20% of the population reported a specific fear of embarrassment while speaking, writing, or eating in public.

In view of the prevalence of speaking anxiety, it is important for concerned professionals to be aware of the progress made in the past two decades in the study of fear and anxiety. The advances made in understanding these phenomena are as exciting and significant as the recent development of instrumentation that enables direct visualization and measurement of laryngeal and brain function. To appreciate how the contemporary understanding and science of anxiety disorders can be applied in SLP clinical practice, fundamental background is needed.

Anxiety Overview

Although most persons have experienced anxiety, its essence has been most vividly captured by great writers. Fear and anxiety might even be considered among the primary elements of narrative drama as a vivid detail in folk tales, myth, plays, and literature throughout history across world cultures. Note Shakespeare's 16th century description of Macbeth:

> Then comes my fit again. I had else been perfect:
> Whole as the marble, founded as the rock,
> As broad and general as the casing air.
> But now I am cabin'd, cribb'd, confin'd, bound in
> To saucy doubts and fears.

> **William Shakespeare, *Macbeth* (Act 3, Scene 4)[2]**

Today, that is called a panic attack.

The Danish existential philosopher, Søren Kierkegaard, wrote about anxiety, labeled "dread," that can be overwhelming:

> And no Grand Inquisitor has in readiness
> Such terrible torture as has dread
> and no spy know how to attack more

[2]From *The Complete Works of Shakespeare* (p. 1308), edited by I. Ribner and G. L. Kittredge, 1971, Waltham, MA: Ginn and Co.

artfully the man he suspects, choosing the
Instant when he is weakest, nor knows how to
lay traps where he will be caught and ensnared,
as dread knows how, and no sharp-witted judge
knows how to interrogate, to examine the
accused as dread does, which never lets him
escape, neither by diversion nor by noise,
neither at work nor at plays, neither by day nor by night.

Søren Kierkegaard, *The Concept of Dread*[3]

This is an apt description of what clinicians label general anxiety disorder (GAD).

Long before Kierkegaard and Shakespeare, the fourth century "father of medicine," Hippocrates, recognized the signs and symptoms of a specific type of anxiety known today as social anxiety, and described an individual who was shy, had a suspicious nature and did not want to be seen in public. The individual feared disgrace and would be sick out of belief that everyone was observing him (Marks, 1969).

Sigmund Freud wrote that the problem of anxiety is "a nodal point at which the most various and important questions converge, a riddle whose solution would be bound to throw a flood of light upon our whole mental existence" (Freud, 1963).

Today, anxiety is viewed as a complex phenomenon of the total response of a human being to threat or danger, imagined or real. It has three components: cognitive, physiological, and behavioral. The cognitive aspect is a persistent, chronic sense of uneasiness or dread from negative perceptions about a present or future event or interchange with a person. The concurrent physiological process of alarm and activation is marked by changes in neural chemistry, among other responses. The behavioral response is often manifested in an emergency fight-or-flight reaction.

Individual variations in interpretation of stimulating events can be seen on worry scales or self-report instruments. These typically measure the cognitive aspect of anxiety as subjective reports of reactions to acts or events. The physiological aspect of anxiety, or arousal, is generally measured by changes in heart rate, respiration, galvanic skin response, muscle tension, body temperature, and cortisol (hydrocortisone) levels. Behavioral reactions can be observed directly or reflected in instruments measuring the type and level of stress, and coping strategies. (See Chapters 3 and 4 for discussion of the affective, cognitive, behavioral, and psychophysiological aspects of anxiety.)

[3]From *The Concept of Dread* (p. 139), by S. Kierkegaard (W. Lowrie, translator), 1944, Princeton, NJ: Princeton University Press.

Perception and reaction to a threat will vary among individuals and situations, ranging from a moment's fleeting concern to a prolonged state of overwhelming anxiety. A situation that may seem benign to many can be a nightmare for an anxious person seized with fear, who fully expects to be harmed. To an anxious person, a triggering event or possibility (such as being asked to speak in a meeting) can lead to high physiological arousal and hypervigilance, loss of focus, and feelings of helplessness and lack of control. Ultimately, an anxious individual becomes trapped in a negative cycle of fear, influenced by a full range of cognitive, physiological, and behavioral effects. Common reactions are avoidance of potentially stressful situations or awkward, self-conscious endurance. Many types of anxiety are universally experienced throughout the lifespan. See Table 1-1.

TABLE 1-1. Common Anxiety Types

Transient Anxiety	Anticipatory Anxiety	State Anxiety	Trait Anxiety
Common phenomenon accompanying life changes, such as separation of children from parents, first dates, new jobs, moving, or loss of loved ones	Surfaces when people dwell on future potential foul-ups	Suffered in a particular situation or with a particular person. Can manifest in any or all of the cognitive, physiological, or behavioral anxiety components.	Individual's typical level of anxiety independent of specific threatening or dreaded environments
Individuals project fears into the future and dwell on potential external catastrophes, with accompanying loss of identity and self-esteem.	Even seasoned speakers, professional musicians, and skilled actors worry incessantly about upcoming performances and fixate on potential catastrophes. This anxiety may or may not disappear during performance.	Fear of certain conversations and public speaking or assertive interactions is a state anxiety for many, who have fear only before performance or when they believe they will be evaluated or observed.	Some have a very high level of trait anxiety, experiencing it internally, even in situations not consciously stressful. Individuals high in trait anxiety are generally blocked in performance and when being evaluated.

Aspects of Anxiety

Anxiety and Arousal

The distinction and relationship between anxiety and arousal (physiological response) is basic to understanding anxiety, generally, and communication apprehension, in particular. It is the rare individual who does not have a physiological response when challenged with performance or evaluation. How these physiological and mental responses to evaluation are managed is key to overcoming performance anxiety.

Anxiety comprises the cognitive and subjective affective reactions to a stressful event that are based on a person's perceptions of the event. If a person is certain that he or she is not understood or clear, the perception of that event will be stressful and result in negative thoughts and embarrassment. Arousal, on the other hand, is the term for the physiological phenomena resulting primarily from the autonomic nervous system's response, such as dry mouth, cold hands, lack of concentration, and hypervigilance. In others words, the subjective perception of an event accompanied by a sense of humiliation triggers objective physiological reactions.

If the physiological arousal response is misunderstood and interpreted as anxiety, a chain reaction is triggered that exacerbates the existing discomfort and adversely affects performance and behavior. For example, just hearing a request to make a toast at a banquet can precipitate shallow breathing and rapid heartbeat, leading to sweating, tightened throat, cold hands, tense muscles, and, ultimately, avoidance of speaking. This frequently happens with people suffering communication apprehension. However, if the physiological arousal is understood and accepted as the body's instantaneous and natural defensive reaction to a perceived threat or challenge, there is generally another outcome: the physiological reactions will diminish, freeing the individual from debilitating hyperarousal. Most important, if the natural arousal to the challenge of a performance is understood, it can be channeled into positive energy and improve the performance.

A number of clinical observations illustrate the powerful influence of negative thinking and feelings (anxiety) on performance. First, people suffering from communication apprehension who take beta-blocking medication to calm down continue to report mental fears. Even persons with paraplegia and little or no autonomic nervous system activity because of spinal cord injuries report feelings of anxiety. Finally, individuals with accelerated heart rates, elevated blood pressure, excessive sweating, and other autonomic arousal symptoms rate their anxiety about performance in the same manner as others who have less physiological symptomology (Marshall, 1994).

Individual Variation

Clearly, one person's challenge can be another's dread. Some people view difficult situations as challenges and cope well. Others react to similar situations devoid of actual danger with intense fear. Such is the case when competent speakers or seasoned actors react as if facing a firing squad or kangaroo court, even when they have a supportive audience. Unfortunately, the mind does not always differentiate between real and imagined fears. Both actual and perceived threats can trigger innate, internal defense mechanisms that result in the same mental and physical anguish. Once a mental alarm is set off in the central nervous system, the body reacts. In communication apprehension, the threat is not physical, but a threat to the sense of personal identity, or self-esteem.

Benefits of Anxiety

Not all anxiety is bad or abnormal. In fact, the concern can be productive and result in emotional growth, if understood and channeled into positive energy. For example, anxiety can motivate people to work hard, to excel, to overcome, or to make money. It is also a lifesaver—an innate survival or defense mechanism that can galvanize a person to recognize and deal with life-threatening situations.

Social Anxiety/Phobia

An anxiety disorder goes beyond normal, transient fears and anxiety. It typically includes heightened sensitivity or the overreaction of a person's internal defense system. Simply thinking of an event believed to be threatening can trigger an autonomic nervous system alarm as demanding as one set off by a real danger. Anxiety disorders are marked by a disabling and chronic process that can disrupt any aspect of life: vocational/professional, academic, social, or familial. There also can be major health consequences as the physiological chemical reactions from prolonged anxiety play havoc with the body's first line of natural defense to disease—the immune system. (See Chapter 3 for details on anxiety and Chapter 4 for a discussion of the psychophysiology of stress.)

In 1980, the publication of the third edition of the *Diagnostic and Statistical Manual of Mental Disorders* (DSM-III; American Psychiatric Association) provided specific definitions of anxiety disorders to be treated through drugs and/or cognitive therapy. At that time anxiety ceased being only a symptom of an underlying unconscious problem. The revised DSM-III (DSM-III-R; American Psychiatric Association, 1987) designated a distinct classification of anxiety disorders known as social phobia. It was defined as a persistent deep fear of one or more situations in which a person is exposed to possible scrutiny by others and fears that he or she may do something resulting in humiliation or embarrassment (see Tables 1-2 and 1-3).

Anxiety disorders have been noted to be the most frequently observed category of emotional disorders in the United States (Leary and Kowalski, 1995). The preponderance of anxiety disorders, especially social anxiety and social phobias, has led to considerable professional interest and research into the subject.

Communication Apprehension: A Type of Social Anxiety/Phobia

In the psychiatric literature, communication apprehension is considered a type of social anxiety. In its extreme form, in which it interferes with an individual's normal daily routines, it is considered a social phobia.

TABLE 1-2. Definition of Social Phobia

Social phobia is a persistent fear of one or more situations in which a person is exposed to possible scrutiny by others and fears that he or she may do something or act in a way that will be humiliating or embarrassing. Social phobia is more than shyness, is common among professional performers, and is treatable.

- Exposure to a specific stimulus generally provokes an anxiety response.
- The feared situation is either avoided or endured with intense anxiety.
- There is marked distress or avoidance behavior that interferes with social and/or occupational functioning.
- There is recognition that one's fear is excessive or unreasonable.

Note. Based on information in *Diagnostic and Statistical Manual of Mental Disorders* (4th ed.), by the American Psychiatric Association. 1994. Washington, DC.

TABLE 1-3. Categories of Social Phobia

Discrete	Generalized
Elicited only by certain situations, such as speaking, performing, eating, or writing in public	Elicited by social situations that involve interpersonal interactions

Ranging from "butterflies in the stomach" to
communication apprehension can disrupt a person's
tion, speech motor processes, and physiological states
a performance. Even the most well-prepared students, executives,
singers, athletes, and actors can become paralyzed by their intense fear
before and during performances.

Signs and Symptoms

Reactions

Physiological signs of communication apprehension include a rise in
the blood levels of neurotransmitters such as epinephrine (adrenalin) or
norepinephrine, blood pressure increases, and body temperature drop.
Data suggest a high level of sympathetic autonomic nervous system
and adrenal gland activation (Taggert, Carruthers, and Somerville as
cited in Marshall, 1994). Respiratory/cardiovascular symptoms before
or during performances include a disturbing self-awareness of accelerated heart rates, blushing, shallow and rapid breathing patterns, light-
headedness accompanied by a fear of fainting, hyperventilation, tremor
or shakiness, weakness in the legs, severe nausea, and sweaty hands.
There can also be a sense or urinary or bowel urgency. Some people can
ignore or channel these autonomic arousal symptoms into positive
energy. However, others—those who can benefit from treatment—are
hypervigilant to their internal cues and cannot tune out their heightened body changes during a performance.

People identified with social phobia were followed in a University of
Wisconsin study as they prepared to present a speech (Marshall, 1994).
An extreme intensity of apprehension was reflected in high activation of
the individuals' right cerebral hemispheres. The process appeared to
interfere with both the logical and verbal preparation of messages, a frequent complaint of speakers—especially those with communication
apprehension.

Fears of performance have little to do with a person's courage, even
the willingness to risk physical danger. For example, a brave firefighter
who feared public speaking more than going into a burning building
said, "I never knew the speech bone was connected to the urinary tract."
Another courageous emergency manager who avoided oral presentations claimed that the terror of public speaking was second only to his
missions as a helicopter pilot in Vietnam. A foreign news correspondent
confessed that he would rather dodge bullets in civil wars than speak in
front of a live audience. Like millions of persons, these people, heroic in
the face of external dangers, cower in front of audiences.

Catastrophic Thoughts

Along with physiological symptoms, communication apprehension that is severe enough to be considered a type of social phobia is accompanied by a cascade of catastrophic thoughts (Beck & Emery, 1985; Daly & Buss, 1984; Paul,1966).

A highly placed executive described his thoughts while speaking, "I feel like my car is about to career off a cliff." Other comments heard frequently before performances included: "I'm going to faint. . . . they're going to know how scared I am. . . . all those eyes are looking at me. . . . I'm going to feel so stupid. . . . I can't get out of this chair, my knees are trembling. . . . I want to bolt." After performing acceptably, people often say, "I have no idea what I said. . . . that was awful. . . . I am so embarrassed." Actually, audiences generally have no idea of the level of discomfort that many performers have and are unaware that a speaker may be fixating on thoughts of appearing ridiculous or weak because of fearfulness.

Characteristics

The characteristics of persons suffering from communication apprehension are detailed in Table 1-4, Characteristics of Communication Anxiety.

Even professionals earning a living from performance can suffer communication anxiety. Interestingly, many have symptoms related to their specific skills. For example, speakers, actors, and singers may have a dry mouth or throat constriction as evidence of stage fright. Athletes and instrumentalists can suffer breakdowns in gross and fine motor skills basic to their musical or athletic ability.

TABLE 1-4. Characteristics of Communication Anxiety

- Intense fears before and during performance
- Heightened physiological arousal (autonomic nervous system and endocrine system reactivity)
- Subjective reactions to arousal (unrelated to intensity of arousal)
- Hypervigilance to bodily reactions
- Sense of loss of control
- Catastrophic thoughts
- Fear of revealing anxiety
- Dread of visual scrutiny
- Fears may not dissipate with experience
- Shift of attention and diffusion of concentration and energy
- Powerful mind-body interrelationship

Breakdowns from anxiety at all levels of skill present powerful evidence of the mind-body connection. This ancient concept implies that a person's every thought, positive and negative, has a physiological response. Therefore, this author believes that every specialist in communications, communication disorders, and the performing arts should be knowledgeable about anxiety and communication apprehension.

Epidemiology

Communication apprehension, especially the fear of speaking in public, has attracted the attention of researchers in psychology, education, business, and entertainment because it is such a common problem. According to the Epidemiological Catchment Area (ECA) study of more than 13,000 Americans (Myers et al., 1984, cited in Schneier, 1993), social phobia, which includes communication apprehension, is a common disorder. The study showed the highest numbers for younger persons (ages 18–29), who are less educated, single, and in a lower socioeconomic class, with a mean onset of 15.5 years.

In a telephone interview of 250 men and 250 women conducted in St. Louis, MO, 21% indicated avoidance of public activities because of embarrassment. Additionally, 21% reported that they had tried to avoid public speaking. Although many people with social phobia are known to have other psychiatric problems, only 5% of persons only having social phobia sought treatment, according to the Harvard Mental Health Letter (Roy-Byrne & Katon, 1994). However, Schneier (1991) reported that, of people seeking treatment for social phobia, at least 30% were male and well educated.

Other surveys have shown that communication apprehension is a major problem among student and professional musicians and actors, who also fear embarrassment during performance. In a study of students and faculty at The University of Iowa School of Music, 16% reported that performance anxiety had limited their careers (Wesner, Noyes, & Davis, cited in Marshall, 1994). In a survey taken at the International Conference of Symphony and Opera Musicians, 24% said they had suffered seriously from stage fright (Roy-Byrne & Katon, 1994). There is also evidence that to varying degrees, the fear of facing an audience is universal, even among some world-class performers whose careers have been interrupted or stopped as a result (Barlow, 1988.) Communication apprehension is, indeed, a serious problem for millions of ordinary and extraordinary people.

Case Examples

A variety of examples of individuals with communication apprehension are presented to illustrate the feelings and behaviors of persons with this problem—some with communication disorders and others with normal speaking ability. This section concludes with examples of professional performers who have also suffered debilitating communication apprehension. These anecdotal reports should vividly convey the impact of this hidden disability on personal and professional lives, along with the potential for success when the problem is treated. First detailed are patients with clearly diagnosed communication disorders and resistance to therapy or difficulty generalizing their learned communication skills. These reports are followed by examples of individuals who are generally competent and articulate communicators when not under stress.

Language Disorder

Ed, a 17-year-old special education student with language impairment was severely limited in reading and writing skills, but had good mechanical ability. His standard language tests scores on overall expressive language ability were slightly below his receptive language, which was low average. Nevertheless, Ed was capable of speaking in intelligible sentences, which were occasionally telegraphic—but completely intelligible.

Although Ed was able to carry on a conversation if the subject was of interest to him, his overall pragmatic language ability (social use of language) including initiating and maintaining conversations with peers and strangers as well as commenting, protesting, requesting, and responding, was very poor. In fact, Ed did not speak up in class, even when he knew the answers to questions. He refused all class outings and spent his days as a social isolate, despite attempts by others to include him in their activities. His functional communication limitations were major obstacles in this young man's social life and vocational potential.

It was only through frequent sessions with the speech clinician that the true nature of Ed's poor pragmatic skills became apparent. He was highly verbal in these sessions and, with help, began to recognize that the source of his withdrawal was his fear of ridicule and embarrassment about speaking. Ed admitted to a sense of panic whenever he had to talk to peers, strangers, or authority figures. He was always reminded of the anguish of his childhood when he was, in fact, slow to develop language. However, his expressive language as a young adult was functional for social and selected vocational purposes. Nevertheless, he scrupulously avoided all situations in which he feared revelation of his weaknesses and the possibility of more humiliation.

Ed was clearly a social phobic, with an inordinate fear of speaking in social and public situations, who was hiding behind and exacerbating his expressive language disorder. No amount of traditional language stimulation would help him overcome this fear, because he was a teenager with all of the other adjustment problems that implies. Ed needed help with his social anxiety and his characteristic coping behavior of avoidance. Only after weeks of discussions and assignments for reducing his fears did Ed take his first field trip, ever, with his class. It was the beginning of a long journey, which has continued.

Fluency Disorders

Clinicians and stutterers alike view the fear of public speaking as solely a consequence of a stuttering problem. However, as Schneier and Welkowitz have shown (1996), many stutterers also suffer from social phobia and would probably be fearful of speaking in public even if they did not stutter. John Alback, an organizer of a self-help group for stutterers, wrote with humor (Alback, 1990) about the fear of humiliation and embarrassment that he suffered when having to address a group of people. It was equal to, if not worse than, the embarrassment he suffered from his dysfluency.

> When I first learned that public speaking was the thing people feared most, I was very surprised. I thought this to be true for those of us who stutter, but not for the public at large. I had always figured that the fear of death would top this list for most people. Upon reflection, however, I came up with three advantages that death has over speaking in front of a group of people. First of all, you are only going to die once, whereas, there is no limit to the number of times you can make a fool of yourself before an audience. Second, death is the best way I know to avoid speaking in front of a group. And, last, but not least, after you die, you do not have to walk back to your seat (p. 13).

Other people who stutter have been helped to recognize the phobic aspect of their speech difficulty and overcome the physiological and cognitive aspects of their social fears. As they confronted and resolved these problems, their stuttering symptoms were no longer an issue. Note the following two cases of Carla and Russ, who entered speech therapy seeking help for their dysfluency.

Carla, a very verbal 32-year-old fund-raiser was convinced that her childhood stuttering problem had returned. She complained that she was beginning to block again on words when she participated in meetings or gave oral presentations to groups, an integral part of her job. She exhibited all of the classic symptoms of hyperarousal associated with performance anxiety, even when thinking about or anticipating a company meeting or a public speaking situation. She experienced a rapid heart rate, shallow breathing and was hypervigilant about her speech and bodily reactions, which she described as "tense." Her normally rapid speech rate accelerated and she rarely paused to replenish her breath when speaking. However, very few of the overt dysfluency symptoms that she complained about were observable during the speech therapy sessions she pursued in an effort to overcome her "speech" problem.

Eventually, Carla understood that the source of her speaking problem was a phobic reaction to specific speaking situations characterized by excessive fear and hyperarousal. She then was helped to modify her cognitive and physiological reactions with anxiety reduction strategies (self-regulation techniques), and her respiratory and cardiac symptoms and bodily tensions abated. No traditional speech therapy techniques were appropriate or necessary in this case of classic communication apprehension. She was dismissed after six therapy sessions.

Russ, a recent college graduate who worked in a prestigious law firm as a paralegal had gone through years of traditional speech therapy beginning in preschool. His most recent speech therapy had focused on the coordination of breathing with phonation and gentle onset, which he had practiced and used diligently. However, his controls failed him on his first job when he had to speak with his superiors. He described his reactions at these times as feeling like his chest was in a vice with his fists clenched (ready for a fight). His fear of speaking to people in his firm escalated as he felt helpless in communicating orally. Although a stutterer, Russ was suffering from a social phobia, a communication apprehension problem that had never been addressed. In eight sessions of therapy that focused on explaining the physiology of speaking anxiety, teaching techniques to reduce his physiological arousal, creating awareness of his distorted thinking, and providing cognitive behavioral strategies to reduce negative thoughts that perpetuated his fears and arousal, Russ's fluency was no longer a problem.

Russ questioned why speech-language pathologists had not previously addressed his phobic reactions or taught him stress management techniques. Several sessions later he stated that he no longer considered himself a stutterer, but rather as a very sensitive person (not weak), who was subject to hyperarousal in situations that he perceived to be threatening, which, in turn, affected his fluency. With help, he quickly learned that his fears, negative thinking, and distorted perceptions of people and events were at the root of his dysfluency and caused his speech controls to break down. Russ no longer needed the speech controls he once relied on after he understood why his fluency broke down in certain situations—the basic problem underlying his episodic stuttering.

Voice Disorders

Veta, an attractive 27-year-old daughter of a mother from a traditional family from India and German father, was convinced that she had a growth on her larynx and insisted that she could not speak louder than a confidential tone. Even though she was reassured by a laryngologist that she had a healthy larynx, she could/would not use a normal conversational voice with others until issues involving her fear of speaking performance were identified and discussed.

Veta was born out of wedlock and was clearly different from her all-Indian siblings in looks, abilities, and ambitions. Her mother had harbored shame about the liaison that had produced Veta and never spoke to her about her biological father. Rather, she continually admonished Veta to be subservient and soft-spoken, all traits typical of a dutiful Indian daughter and wife.

Desperate to get away, Veta broke with her cultural background, worked her way through college despite the ridicule of her uneducated siblings, and eventually married a supportive Irish-American man. She was working as a secretary with ambitions to return to graduate school, but realized she would have problems unless she did something about her voice. Everyone, especially at work, complained that they could neither hear nor understand her. Veta was convinced that she had a tumor on her larynx, because she could not speak louder no matter how hard she tried. Finally, she sought professional help.

It was only after an examination by a laryngologist, who reassured her about the health of her larynx, and explanations of the vocal instrument by a speech-language pathologist that she learned to control her vocal intensity (volume). Following an exploration of the mind-body connection and a discussion of her problem, Veta realized the source of her vocal difficulty. She understood, for the first time, the powerful effect her (hidden) fear of being heard had on her voice production. Veta suffered the terror and shame of being found out when speaking, a symptom of communication apprehension. Her mind and body were locked in a heated struggle about speaking up, being heard, and being herself. After six sessions, Veta used her voice normally, even shouting when necessary. The culmination of this dramatic turn of events was a trip to Germany in search of her paternal roots.

Jeanette, a trained opera singer with a coloratura voice, was seeing her laryngologist for voice therapy because of slight right vocal fold fullness, arytenoid erythema, and muscular tension. No glottic closure was noted on certain pitches. Jeannette had stopped pursuing her professional career because of her voice problem, worked as a typist, and only sang in a church choir on weekends. Her restricted vocal range and inability to control her volume devastated her. She could not even call her dog in the same melodic way to which she was accustomed. She stated that the pitch of her speaking voice had lowered, which, in turn, affected her singing voice.

Jeannette reported that her problem had begun in college after she had broken up with her boyfriend of many years. Although she was in psychotherapy and had learned a great deal about herself, she was still unable to sing. She believed that her unhappiness was "choking her" and that even her laugh was "locked in." Further questioning revealed that Jeannette had suffered panic attacks in high school and, although those episodes abated, she complained of emotional lability and shallow breathing. She was petrified about singing solos in church and could not tolerate even the thought of singing alone to an audience, especially "Ava Maria," which had a profound emotional effect on her.

Visibly anxious, Jeannette knew little about the vocal mechanism, especially for a trained singer, and even less about the mind-body connection. Discussion about the psychophysiological effects of fear on the respiratory and cardiovascular systems and muscle tonus as well as the relationship between perceived fears, negative thoughts, and physiological reactions, answered many of this patient's questions about her emotional lability and physical symptoms. Jeannette learned self-regulation strategies to control her physiological reactions, especially through slow diaphragmatic breathing. She also engaged in visual imagery with a hand-held biofeedback instrument that measured the effects of her autonomic system reactivity. This enabled her to recognize and release her laryngeal-pharyngeal tensions as she sang, spoke, and laughed. Jeannette regained her full phonational range, was able to sing solo in church, call her dog in her usual and melodic way, and resumed her professional career.

Normal Speakers—No Disorder

The vast majority of people who suffer from communication apprehension have no complaints of speech, voice, or language disorders and are generally competent and articulate speakers when not under stress. However, in certain situations, or with specific people, they become frozen with fear, as if they were disabled speakers.

Marjorie, a bright, dynamic, and experienced speech-language pathologist, worked in the New York City school system with children with speech and language disorders. However, despite the urging of her principal and speech supervisor, she adamantly refused to conduct groups or classes for parents or teachers because she "simply could not do it." Marjorie openly stated that she had been afraid of any kind of public performance since childhood and that many years of psychotherapy had done nothing to reduce her painful and embarrassing communication anxiety.

Seeking help for this problem was a big step for Marjorie, who could no longer tolerate her own avoidance behavior. She enrolled in a course to overcome her speaking fears. She knew that she had to change and change she did after she recognized the effects of some very destructive messages she received when growing up. Messages such as: "You must be perfect," "You will never succeed," "Who do you think you are?" and other equally demeaning remarks had convinced her that she was unworthy, helpless, and subject to harsh judgments from others.

Gradually, through a systematic program of cognitive restructuring, physiological monitoring, desensitization, and affective support from her peers in reappraising her misperceptions of herself and her power, Marjorie changed. Presently, she is volunteering to run meetings for neighborhood committees and conducting parent and teacher groups in her school, an integral part of her job responsibility.

Ren, a 40-year-old accountant from a traditional Chinese background was raised in Singapore, had a strict parochial school education, and was the only one of five children to come to the United States. Although she had been in the United States for 20 years, she recognized that her inability to interact comfortably with people, to make small talk as well as to speak up in public, was extremely detrimental to her personal and professional advancement. As a result, she felt extremely frustrated, isolated, and depressed about her situation.

Ren described her early background as extremely punitive. Although she had many ideas, she rarely spoke at home or in school as a child. After class discussions of possible reasons for speaking fears, Ren's insights were sharpened and the reasons for her lifelong avoidance of speaking became obvious to her. She then was able to share the experiences of her early years in a strict parochial school where she was frequently "whacked" by the nuns for venturing independent opinions. Afterwards, when she told her parents about her school problems, she was "again whacked" for getting into trouble at school. Although Ren complained about not being able to speak in social or professional situations, she was by far the most outspoken student in a class of 18, all of whom were terrified of performing in public. It was as if she had finally found a forum where she could release her unnatural and self-imposed silence.

Ren made dramatic progress after she presented several presentations in front of the group. The desensitization procedures, feedback, and videotapings helped her to see herself as others saw her, thereby dispelling the misperceptions she had of herself. Before the 8-week class was over, Ren interviewed for a new job in a very competitive industry, impressed the employer, and received a job offer—something she was certain she could not have done a few weeks earlier.

Professional Performers with Performance Anxiety

Many people are amazed to learn that some very talented and famous professional performers suffer severe performance anxiety, or communication apprehension, even years after they have reached the pinnacle of their success.

Actors. According to Stephan Aaron (1986) in *Stage Fright: Its Role in Acting,*

> The actor's conscious fear is not that he will make a mistake but that the audience will see something it is not supposed to see, namely his fear, his stage fright. It is not simply the fear of being seen or breaking the fantasy of the character being portrayed but rather being seen as absurd (p. 59).

This is the same debilitating fear suffered by nonprofessionals, also a form of social phobia.

Sir Laurence Olivier, regarded by many as one of the greatest actors of the last century, wrote openly about his lifelong struggle with stage fright. He compared stage fright to "an animal, a monster which hides in its foul corner without revealing itself, but you know that it is there and that it may come forward at any moment"(Olivier, 1986, p. 181).

At the age of 57, Olivier wrote in his autobiography about his first bout with terror, which occurred when he was 13. It was after his beloved mother's death, a year before, when he was singing in the choir for which she had trained him. He wrote: "My breath left my body and could not be retrieved; my throat closed up and I was forced to stop" (Olivier, 1982, p. 261–262).

He later wrote:

> These crises were unpredictably sporadic and have been a nightmare to me all my life in public appearance. . . . It is always waiting outside the door, any door, waiting to get

you. You either battle or walk away . . . suddenly there he is, the bogeyman comes along and tries to rob you of your living. He can come at any time, in any form . . . the dark shadow of fear . . . Just when you think you've conquered it, and there it is sitting at the end of the bed grinning at you (Olivier, 1986, p. 180–183).

Olivier's remedy for his stage fright was to give instructions to the other actors not to look him in the eyes, something completely antithetical to good acting. He admitted that for some reason this made him feel that there was not quite so much loaded against him.

Joyce Ashley, Jungian and psychoanalyst, who espouses a Jungian view of stage fright, believed that Olivier's reaction was an outgrowth of the frequent corporal punishment to which he was subjected as a child and young man. According to his sisters, the father had been very severe with young Laurence, the last of four children, and took his rage out on him physically. Ashley (1996) interpreted Olivier's stage fright remedy of having fellow actors lower their eyes or avert their gaze and related it to the feelings of shame Olivier suffered from the corporal punishment he was forced to endure in his formative years. Lowering the eyes and gaze aversion are well-known signs of shame and a central element in communication apprehension.

Olivier was notoriously averse to introspection and never treated his panic other than by self-medicating with alcohol and, finally, Valium. He believed later that his stage fright "simply wore itself out," but, in fact, his final years were marked by serious and painful illnesses. According to Ashley, somehow, his psychological pain found expression in his body. Although Olivier was unable to constructively overcome his private hell, he was able to illuminate the devastating feelings of a famous performer caught in a demonic web and his ambivalent relationship with an audience:

When the actor is on stage, it is he and he alone who drives the moment. The audience has no choice but to remain in his faith or leave. That's the true excitement, the real magic of the profession. The actor on stage is all-powerful, for once the curtain rises, he is in control. . . .Without them (the audience) you do not exist. Without them you are a man alone in a room with memories and a mirror. Without them you are nothing (Olivier, 1986, p. 369–370).

Other famous performers, who did not have difficult upbringings, also have spoken freely of their continual struggle with stage fright, even after hundreds of anxiety-free performances.

Maureen Stapleton describes her stage fright, which has a distinctive and confounding symptom, especially when persisting during a performance. She has reported, "when I work, it starts about 6:30 at night. I start to burp. I belch, almost nonstop. I keep burping, all through the show, right up to the curtain, and right after, and then I'm all right" (Marshall, 1944, p. 141).

Gertrude Laurence, a great stage comedian and performer, remarked, "These attacks of nerves seem to grow worse with the passing of the years. It's inexplicable and horrible and something you'd think you'd grow out of, not into" (Marshall, 1994, p. 33).

Rosalind Russell, an acting diva, has said cryptically, "Acting is like standing up naked and turning around very slowly" (Marshall, 1994, p. 134). Implicit in that statement is the potential for humiliation in being fully revealed, naked, unmasked, and scrutinized.

Musicians. The virtuoso pianist, Vladimir Horowitz, quit performing for 15 years and was nearly incapacitated by anxiety when he did manage to resume performing. He had a recurring dream that his fingers would turn to glass. Arthur Rubinstein, Pablo Casals, and Luciano Pavarotti have all reported extreme performance anxiety. Casals said, "Nerves and stage fright before playing have never left me throughout the whole of my career" (Corredor, 1956, p. 29). Carly Simon placed her career on hold for 6 years after collapsing in front of 10,000 people because of her fear. Barbra Streisand has been very open about her struggles with performance anxiety. She has been able to perform at charity and political functions, but was unable to perform as a paid artist for 27 years. Perhaps this is because she feels that paying audiences may be more critical or judgmental (Marshall, 1994).

Athletes. Even athletes who employ gross motor skills in such sports as baseball suffer serious disruptions from performance anxiety. Mike Ivie, a highly promising young catcher for the San Diego Padres, became so phobic about throwing the ball back to the pitcher that he had to give up his position. Steve Sax, a second baseman for the Los Angeles Dodgers, was unable to make routine throws to first base; Steve Blass, the Pittsburgh Pirate World Series hero and all-star pitcher, mysteriously and suddenly could not get the ball over the plate in a game in 1973, although he had been able to do so perfectly in practice. The anxiety ended his career at the age of 32. New York Mets catcher Mickey Sasser, a talented and highly paid left-handed catcher, could not return the ball to the mound without going through a bizarre routine. This occurred only when people were watching him and cost him his job. These athletes were all suffering aspects of social phobia.

The list of professional performers, actors, singers, musicians, and athletes who suffer from performance anxiety is endless. Despite years of training and experience performing in public, the performance anxiety of rich and famous celebrities is just as intense as ordinary citizens playing a role on the stage of life. These performers are classic examples of the intimate relationship between the mind and the body. Training, experience, even years of success could not diminish the terror of these talented people.

Professional Concerns and Opportunities

Although communication disorder specialists acknowledge that anxiety is a factor in many problems they treat, communication apprehension has been ignored as a disorder or even as an area of professional concern. This neglect is understandable for several reasons. First, there is a lack of awareness of the prevalence, seriousness and consequences of the problem. Second, speech-language pathologists generally do not treat "non-pathological" conditions and anxiety and communication apprehension, a psychophysiological phenomenon, is not considered an organic problem. Furthermore, like stuttering, the problem is episodic and context-dependent, and most people with speaking anxiety neither discuss it nor seek help. Unfortunately, school speech-language pathologists, who are in the best position to assist teachers identify and help youngsters with incipient communication apprehension, and university speech and communications departments who can easily offer services or courses focus on more obvious communication disorders.

The neglect of communication apprehension by communication disorder specialists is a conundrum because, although the effect of physical stress on vocal performance is always considered, the psychophysiological reactions from stress or evaluation on communication performance is not systematically addressed. This presents problems for vocologists, in particular, who often complain about the lack of transfer and maintenance of normal voice after working effectively with patients in the clinic. Such was the case with a transgender professor who reportedly was successful at establishing a feminine voice in the clinic, but could not project or transfer her new voice in the classroom (personal communication, Doug Hicks, May 21, 1999). Similarly, a Jewish cantor who was successfully treated for a voice problem from nodules resulting from vocal abuse was unable to maintain his voice during religious performances.

He was too scared. Discussion with the clinician of the latter client indicated that she did not know how to deal with his stage fright although she was aware of the problem (personal communication, Amy Rader, June 1998). This situation occurs with other speech and language problems as well, as illustrated in this chapter's case examples. Finally, some voice and speech patients may be considered malingerers when no organic basis for their problem is found. This is unfortunate, because many patients with symptoms, but no pathophysiology, may be suffering somatization of their anxieties, a problem that appears to be increasing in primary care practices (Barsky & Borus, 1995), as well as voice clinics (personal communication, Doug Hicks, May 21, 1999).

Neglecting or underestimating the effects of communication apprehension and anxiety on patients can lead to a misdiagnosis or unsuccessful treatment of a disorder. Standard diagnostic instrumentation and tests alone do not reflect the effects of mental stress or worry on performance. Nor does any amount of training on oral or laryngeal musculature, intensive language stimulation, or desensitization procedures alone address the problems of communication apprehension. It is essential that a whole person be treated, not just a disorder.

Rationale for Treating Communication Apprehension

Communication apprehension, a psychophysiological disorder, is suffered by a huge untapped population who could be effectively treated by speech-language pathologists. These people suffer anguish and consequences as serious as some who stutter or have other communication disorders. Communication apprehension is also a problem for many patients with clearly diagnosed communication disorders. A relationship between social phobia and some stutterers already has been found (Schneier and Welkowitz, 1996). Moreover, Menzies, Onslow and Packman (1999) reviewed the literature on anxiety and stuttering and found it woefully inadequate, causing a serious problem, both academically and clinically. They called for more examination of the issues. It stands to reason that understanding about the psychophysiology of anxiety (see Chapters 3 and 4), which is so apparent in persons who do not stutter, will lead to a greater understanding of the effects of anxiety on all communication disorder patients, especially those who stutter. The problem of communication apprehension is a legitimate concern for communication disorder specialists, who have much to offer those who suffer from the problem.

There are also practical reasons why speech-language pathologists should treat communication anxiety. Most significantly, they have as comprehensive a background as any professionals in allied fields to treat this problem, having been trained in the science and biology of communication and communication disorders, behavioral management, and communication skills. With some additional training in the origins and management of anxiety and communication apprehension, SLPs can develop their expertise, broaden their armamentarium, and enlarge their scope of practice. In addition, SLPs are probably the most acceptable professionals to work with this population, because they have the best understanding of the skills, demands, and needs of speakers and performing artists.

Interestingly, there are few places that offer the kind of comprehensive help needed by those suffering from communication apprehension, especially when it involves speaking. A hospital setting or psychiatric clinic is hardly conducive to someone who fears speaking or performing in public, especially if they have a discrete or circumscribed problem. Speech-language pathologists are already in educational settings where the problem can be easily identified. This holds true for performing artist mentors in schools of music and drama. School SLPs, university speech clinics and Performing Arts Departments can easily include substantive performance anxiety programs in their curricula. Professional colleagues, such as psychologists and psychiatrists, can always be used as consultants or collaborators, as necessary.

Finally, attention to mind-body issues and the inclusion of systematic anxiety assessment and anxiety reduction strategies can help put the whole person back into the treatment of all communication disorders. It can also enhance the performance of every professional performer. Anxiety, after all, involves the central and autonomic nervous systems, affecting cognition, respiration, physiology, muscle tonus, affect, and behavior, all of which are involved in a person's ability to communicate, vocalize, speak, and perform effectively.

Chapter Summary

Communication apprehension is a pervasive, multifaceted phenomenon that must be viewed from many perspectives if it is to be understood and overcome. It is a psychophysiological problem that has been neglected by the communication disorders profession, which should strive to include the study of mind-body issues, in general, and performance anxiety, in particular. Understanding and treating communication apprehension, whatever it is called, is beneficial to patients as well as specialists concerned with effective communication performance.

Chapter 2 discusses the development of social and performance anxiety from various perspectives.

References

Aaron, S. (1986). *Stage fright: Its role in acting*. Chicago: University of Chicago Press.

Alback, J. (1990). *To say what is ours: The best ten years of letting go*. San Francisco: National Stuttering Project.

American Psychiatric Association. (1980). *Diagnostic and statistical manual of mental disorders* (3rd ed.). Washington, DC: Author.

American Psychiatric Association. (1987). *Diagnostic and statistical manual of mental disorders* (3rd ed., rev.). Washington, DC: Author.

American Psychiatric Association. (1994). *Diagnostic and statistical manual of mental disorders* (4th ed.). Washington, DC: Author.

Ashley, J. (1996). *Overcoming stage fright in everyday life*. NY: Clarkson Potter.

Barlow, D. H. (1988). *Anxiety and its disorders*. NY: Guilford Press.

Barsky, A. J. & Borus, J. F. (1995, December 27). Somatization and medicalization in the era of managed care. *Journal of the American Medical Association, 274*, 1931–1934.

Beck, A. T. & Emery, G. (1985). *Anxiety disorders and phobias: A cognitive perspective*. NY: Basic Books.

Buss, A. (1984). A conception of shyness. In J. A. Daly & J. C. McCroskey (Eds.), *Avoiding communication: Shyness, reticence, and communication apprehension* (pp. 34–39). Beverly Hills, CA: Sage Publications.

Buss, A. H. (1980). *Self-consciousness and social anxiety*. San Francisco: W. H. Freeman.

Corredor, J. M. (1956). *Conversations with Casals*. NY: Dutton.

Daly, J. A. & Buss, A. H. (1984). The transitory causes of audience anxiety. In J. A. Daly & J. C. McCroskey (Eds.), *Avoiding communication: Shyness, reticence, and communication apprehension* (pp. 67–68). Beverly Hills, CA: Sage Publications.

Edelman, R. J. (1992). *Anxiety: Theory, research and intervention in clinical and health psychology*. Chichester: NY: John Wiley.

Everly, G. S. Jr. & Rosenfeld, R. (1981). *The nature and treatment of the stress response: A practical guide for clinicians*. NY: Plenum Press.

Feldman, L. (1991, July 7). Strikeouts and psych-outs. *New York Times Magazine*, 10–13, 30.

Freud, S. (1963). *The problem of anxiety* (H. A. Bunker, Trans.). NY: Psychoanalytic Quarterly Press.

Hickerson, J. C. (1997). *A biofeedback/cognitive-behavioral treatment model for women with public speaking anxiety*. Unpublished doctoral dissertation, University of Texas, Arlington.

Holbrook, H. T. (1987). *Communication apprehension: The quiet student in your classroom.* (ERIC Digest No. Ed 284315). Urbana, IL: ERIC Clearinghouse on Reading and Communication Skills. Retrieved October 2, 2000 from ERIC database (No. ED 284315), available at: http://www.ed.gov/databases/ERIC_Digests/ed284315.html

Leary, M. & Kowalski, R. (1995). *Social anxiety.* NY: The Guilford Press.

Marks, I. M. (1969). *Fears and phobias.* NY: Academic Press.

Marshall, J. (1994). *Social phobia: From shyness to stage fright.* New York: Basic Books.

Menzies, R., Onslow, M., & Packman, A. (1999). Anxiety and stuttering: Exploring a complex relationship. *American Journal of Speech and Hearing Research, 8*, 3–10.

Miller, S. & Watson, B. C. (1992). The relationship between communication attitude, anxiety, and depression in stutterers and nonstutterers. *Journal of Speech and Hearing Research, 35*, 789–798.

Olivier, L. (1982). *Confessions of an actor: An autobiography.* NY: Simon and Schuster.

Olivier, L. (1986). *Laurence Olivier on acting.* NY: Simon and Schuster.

Paul, G. (1966). *Insight versus desensitization in psychotherapy: An experiment in anxiety reduction.* Palo Alto, CA: Stanford University Press.

Peavey, B. (1995, November). *Fear and fluency: The physiology of arousal and speech production.* Short course presented at the annual convention of the American Speech-Language-Hearing Association, Orlando, FL.

Pollard, C. A. & Henderson, J. G. (1988). *Four types of social phobia in a community sample,* The Journal of Nervous and Mental Disease, Vol. 176, No. 7, p. 440–445.

Roy-Byrne, P. & Katon, W. (1994, November). An update on tx of anxiety disorders: Social phobia—Part II. *Harvard Mental Health Letter, 11*, No. 5, p. 1–3.

Schneier, F. R. (1993). The diagnosis, etiology and management of social phobias. *Directions in Psychiatry, 13*, No. 6, p. 1–6.

Schneier, F., Johnson, J., Hornig, D., Liebowitz, M., & Weissman, M. (1992). Social phobia, comorbidity and morbidity in an epidemiologic sample. *Archives of General Psychiatry, 49*, 282–288.

Schneier, F., & Welkowitz, L. (1996). *The hidden face of shyness: Understanding and overcoming social anxiety.* NY: Avon Books.

Schneier, F. R., Wexler, K. B., & Liebowitz, M. R. (1997). Social phobia and stuttering. *American Journal of Psychiatry, 154*, 131.

Slipman, S. (1986). *Helping ourselves to power.* NY: Pergamon.

Stein, M., Baird, A., & Walker, J. (1996). Social phobia in adults with stuttering. *American Journal of Psychiatry, 153*, 278–280.

CHAPTER

2

Developmental Perspectives

o set the stage for comprehending communication apprehension, it is important to understand the bases of fear and anxiety in general, that is, how and why it develops in humans. This chapter addresses the following fundamental questions pertaining to those issues.

1. Is the brain wired to predispose humans to fear certain situations?
2. Why do people fear social and speaking situations?
3. Why are some people predisposed to suffer anxiety—particularly communication anxiety?
4. What role does learning play in the development of communication apprehension?
5. How does culture influence the etiology and maintenance of communication apprehension?

The chapter concludes with a discussion of other factors that may precipitate and/or perpetuate communication apprehension.

Is the Brain Wired to Predispose Humans to Fear Certain Situations?

Viewpoints over the Years

The nature of emotions, especially fear and its relationship to thought, has been debated for centuries. In pondering the question, William James, the nineteenth-century American philosopher, compared the genuine life-threatening dangers from predators endured by our early ancestors to the fears suffered by his contemporaries (cited in Thompson, 1988). James noted that, in spite of the relative safety of his world, people continued to have strong fear reactions. The Jamesian line of thought led to the notion that fear may be an innate evolutionary aspect of our species—and that perception of threats associated with danger (whatever its nature) results in stress responses. Interestingly, vast fear industries that stimulate fear, such as spooky theme parks, scary rides, and creepy motion pictures and novels, are popular and lucrative. It is as if an archival survival circuit in the brain is activated and titillated when simulated threatening events are experienced. More serious than the popular entertainment of fear, there has been a proliferation of anxiety disorders—especially social phobias—even in children. Because of this increase in anxiety disorders, research has focused on the anatomy of fear.

Experiments exploring the fear circuitry in the brains of other animals have been followed by brain imaging studies on humans with anxiety disorders. Every aspect of fear is being scrutinized, measured, recorded, and mapped in the brain. Computerized tomography (CT) images illustrate the brain areas that become active when subjects are presented with fearful stimuli. By coupling these neurological insights with recent findings in such cognitive phenomena as memory, major advances in understanding all emotional phenomena, especially fear, have been made in the last half century (Kagan, 1994).

Fear Circuitry in the Brain

Human and nonhuman animal brain studies have verified that the **amygdala**, a tiny brain area near the brainstem, is the source of fear. Recent experiments have shown that fear travels along at least two

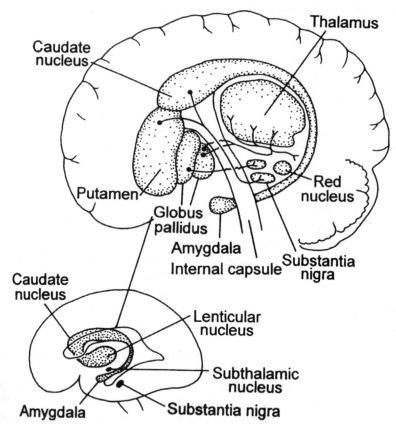

FIGURE 2-1. Location of the amygdala within the Limbic System.

distinct pathways in the brain (Hall, 1999). One pathway threads its way through the higher cortical parts of the brain, believed to be the home of higher thought and then travels to the amygdala. The other pathway, which is very rapid, is just below the level of awareness and rapidly courses to the amygdala.

Located in the lower portion of the brain that links with the spinal cord, the amygdala belongs to the portion of the brain also found in reptiles and birds, as well as mammals that evolved before humans. It is part of the limbic system, which has long been associated with emotion, especially fear (Hall, 1999). The amygdala is shown in Figure 2-1.

Kapp, Pascoe, and Bixler (1984) and LaDoux (1994a), two major researchers of fear, have identified the amygdala, especially its central sulcus, as the seat of fear in the brains of nonhuman animals. They have also shown that nerve fibers from the amygdala project into the upper brain regions that control the release of stress hormones, which play major roles in human irrational fears (see Table 2-1). Therefore, when a person perceives a threat, alarms go off in the brain, causing arousal, hypervigilance, and a host of other autonomic nervous system reactions. The reaction is known clinically as the stress response, or the fight-or-flight response, illustrated in Figure 2-2. The autonomic reactions also result in what is termed the "creeping death" by nervous speakers as they anticipate their turn to make a presentation. (See Chapters 3 and 4 for further discussion of this dynamic.)

TABLE 2-1. Pathway and Effects of Messages From the Amygdala*

Target in Brain of Amygdalic Message	Functional Result	How Measured
Lateral hypothalamus	Sympathetic activity	Changes in heart rate, galvanic skin response, pupil size, blood pressure
Dorsal motor nucleus of vagus	Parasympathetic activity	Ulcers, urination and defacation, decrease in heart rate
Parabrachial nucleus of the pons	Increased respiration	Panting, respiratory distress
Locus ceruleus; ventral tegmentum	Production of norepinephrine	Behavioral arousal, vigilance, EEG activation
Nucleus reticularis pontis caudalis in medulla	Increased vigor of reflexes	Startle
Central gray	Cessation of behavior	Freezing
Trigeminal and facial motor	Movements of the mouth and jaw	Facial expression of fear
nerve Paraventricular nucleus of the hypothalamus	Release of ACTH from the pituitary	Increased cortisol

(Adapted from "The Role of the Amygdala in Fear and Anxiety," by M. Davis, 1992, *Annual Review of Neuroscience*, 15, p. 356. Copyright 1992 by Annual Reviews: Palo Alto, CA. Adapted with permission.)

*This table shows how messages from the amygdala to other parts of the brain (targets) result in physical responses (consequences) that can be measured.

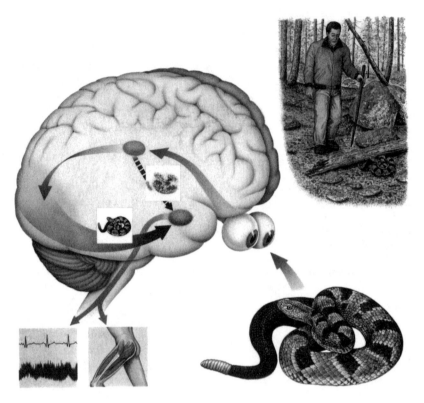

FIGURE 2-2. Fear response.

The fear response evoked when seeing a snake on a path begins with visual stimuli initially processed by the thalamus, which directs basic, nearly archetypal, information straight to the amygdala. This nearly instantaneous spurt promotes rapid brain response to potential danger. At the same time, the visual cortex processes the same information with more refinement, with the more precise details then relayed to the amygdala, causing increases in heart rate and blood pressure, along with muscle contraction. (From "Emotion, Memory, and the Brain," by J. E. LaDoux, 1994, *Scientific American, 270,* p. 38. Copyright 1994 by *Scientific American.* Reprinted with permission.)

Unconscious Fear Activation

LaDoux's work with rats (1994b) has shown that it takes only 12 milliseconds (12 one-thousandth of a second) for a shock to travel from the ear to the lateral nucleus of the amygdala. At that fear center, the cells "learn and memorize" the pain and a fearful response. The stimulus is processed with incredible speed and is imprinted with tenacity. LaDoux's research suggests that it takes only one terrifying experience for a lifelong emotional memory to be put into place that is extremely difficult to erase, because the "thinking" part of the brain is "out of the loop" when the fear-related memory is formed. It further suggests that many fearful situations are experienced, learned, and unconsciously committed to emotional memory without people being aware of the initial fear trigger. This is the source of a true panic attack in which victims are unaware of the source of their overreactions. (See Figure 2-2.)

Lack of cause-and-effect awareness is also typical of many who have performance anxiety. Not being able to pinpoint the cause of their fear leads to a feeling of being weak and helpless. Because the fear is probably lurking in the amygdala and is not connected to conscious memory, groping for the actual source of the fear is generally useless.

Evidence from neuroimaging labs also supports the suggestions from nonhuman animal experiments that fear circuitry can be activated without awareness of the fearful stimulus (Kagan, 1994; LaDoux, 1994b). The evidence also supports the view that fear and anxiety can form unconsciously and bypass the cognitive (thinking) portion of the brain. Further evidence of the unconscious nature of the fear system is that it can be activated through words, hearsay, rumor, subliminal suggestion, empathy with someone else's fears, and even by audiotapes or videotapes of critical parents.

The brain is a vigilant system that becomes hypervigilant whenever a sense of impending danger is evoked, resulting in a chain of psychophysiological events that seems to spiral out of control for those held in the sway of its effects. The symptoms of these events are a manifestation of the body's innate defense system against danger, whether real or perceived.

Anxiety Disorders and the Prefrontal Orbital Cortex

Jack Gorman, a researcher (quoted in Hall, 1999) who has been studying anxiety disorders for 20 years, believes that each variation of anxiety disorder, including phobias, represents a "glitch" somewhere in the fear circuitry, either because of an inherited biochemistry (nature) or a remembered experience (nurture). All of this, in turn, is modulated by the effects of stress, which alters body chemistry in a way that accentuates irrational fears and by the effects of cognition (thoughts), which can either create or defuse irrational fears.

Gorman was also quoted as believing (Hall, 1999) that anxiety disorders, a uniquely human phenomenon, involve the prefrontal cortex, the part of the brain that differentiates us from the chimpanzees. This is in agreement with the trailblazing work of Allan Schore (Schore, 1994), who points out that the prefrontal orbital cortex is a crucial regulator of emotions and motivational and social behavior, as well as the autonomic nervous system. Schore states that the prefrontal orbital cortex can easily malfunction, either because of faulty or traumatic interactions between infant and caregiver or as a result of genetic problems. This implies that very early experiences, even in infants, can be indelibly implanted in the minds and chemistry of people, affecting their reactions to stress over a lifetime. Therefore, the orbitofrontal cortex also plays a major role in the acquisition and evocation of fear.

Schore concluded that consciousness, usually thought to connote only cognitive processes, has an essential affective component. Hence, in addition to the circuitry of conscious and unconscious fears through the amygdala and its connections, the orbitofrontal cortex also plays a major role in the acquisition and evocation of fear. The point is that most of what the brain does occurs outside of awareness and is generally inaccessible without therapy of some sort. The following cases illustrate the power of the unconscious and its relationship to communication anxiety.

Case Examples: Actualized Problems of Unconscious Fears

George, a successful art director in an advertising agency exemplifies how an unconscious fear that spiraled out of control was activated by an association with an old fearful memory. George scrupulously avoided speaking in meetings or groups and did not understand the source of his overwhelming anxiety. Desperate to overcome his problem, he enrolled in the class, Speaking Without Fear, because he wanted to advance in his career, something he understood required communicating in groups. However, during the first session he fled when it came close to his time to introduce himself to the group. He remained in the bathroom until the end of the session. Afterward, in a discussion with the instructor, he realized that the very presence of a woman leading the group brought back a flood of memories about his punitive first grade teacher in a strict parochial school. Apparently he was a high-spirited, or rambunctious, child who exasperated the teacher. In an effort to teach him a lesson about being quiet, she sat him on her desk and placed a dunce cap on his head, with a placard around his neck that read "Dunce." Mortified by this experience, this normally outgoing, creative youngster learned his lesson well. He never spoke up in any class or group again!

Although George did not recall the specifics of that school incident some 30 years previously until he was encouraged to talk about it with the instructor, his body remembered the fear and humiliation that he endured as a child when speaking in a group. The speech class in which he enrolled to overcome his unresolved fear immediately conjured up his repressed first grade memory and triggered old, painful feelings. For this reason, he bolted from the class. George was unable to continue with the course because of the intensity of his fears. He was referred to a psychiatrist for help.

Another example of a person who experienced the unleashing of an unconscious fear is Nancy, whose problem was successfully resolved. She was a gregarious writer who panicked when she was told by her publisher that she would have to go on tour to promote her first book. This tour required her to speak about her book to various audiences, something she had scrupulously avoided throughout her successful academic life, electing instead to express herself in writing. Like George, she never understood the reason for her fear until she completed some thought-provoking homework and participated in group discussions as part of the Speaking Without Fear class in which she had enrolled as a last resort to overcome her fear.

Eventually, Nancy recalled a very embarrassing experience she had endured as a kindergarten student. An audience had laughed at her performance as a dwarf in a school production of *Snow White and the Seven Dwarfs*. Alarmed and humiliated by the laughter, probably provoked because she looked so adorable, she ran offstage and had not stopped running from spoken performances until she recalled the actual precipitating event of her communication apprehension. The turnaround in Nancy's behavior was dramatic. Once the curtain shielding her fear was lifted, she became an outspoken class leader and excellent speaker. Subsequently, she engaged in many successful speaking tours about her book and was a guest on 27 live television shows to promote it.

The stories of George and Nancy exemplify research implications that humans have a separate memory of fearful stimuli lodged in the amygdala, probably informed by things that have been seen or heard, but not consciously remembered. These fears are generally inaccessible because they are unconscious anxieties and outside of awareness. Fear seems to have a long shelf life in the cells where memory is warehoused. It is forever soldered in the circuitry, waiting for the right circumstance to again trigger an avoidance effect. The trigger could be words, hearsay, rumor, subliminal suggestion, or even empathy for someone else's fear. (See Jill case example later in the chapter.)

Cortical Connection of Worry

Davis of Emory University (1992) investigated the high road approach to the processing of fear in humans, which is similar to routine information processing in humans. He found that signals from the sensory organs (such as eyes and ears) linger in the cortex, where conscious memories are formed, before going to a portion of the amygdala. He proposed that these signals control chronic states of fear, such as human anxiety and worry. Unlike humans, other animals have more instinctual fears and lack the capacity to worry about the future or imagine the worst.

Case Example: Worry and Communication Apprehension

The worry and fear of many people about performance can be transformed, or somatized, into physical symptoms, which exacerbates their communication anxieties. This phenomenon is clear in the case of Virginia, a 35-year-old former computer programmer, who was promoted to a supervisory position. Her position required that she conduct frequent training sessions, something she fixated on and dreaded. As a result, she suffered severe neck and back pains 2 days before and after her presentations. She was in good health and had not previously had any such physical complaints. Virginia had never connected her physical symptoms to the fear she felt about speaking in public until she discussed it with the instructor of the class she enrolled in to overcome her performance anxiety. Her tensions and worry were somatized (manifested physically). Her body responded to her unconscious message of danger, a powerful indication of the mind-body connection, something she had never realized before. Once she understood the source of her muscle tension and addressed the irrationality of her negative thoughts and misperceptions about presentations, Virginia's pain abated.

Effects of Medication and Cognitive-Behavioral Therapy on Brain Fear Wiring

Other evidence of the wiring of the brain for fear comes from the positive effects that drugs and cognitive-behavioral therapy have on anxiety. Drugs and cognitive-behavioral therapy apparently override the effects of the amygdala. According to Marshall (1994) drugs prescribed for anxiety reduction seem to work by blocking the molecules that arouse the fear circuitry. Inderal, a beta-blocker, used for communication, performance, and other anxiety works by blocking signals (or messages) from the sympathetic branch of the autonomic nervous system that cause physical symptoms. Drugs have even been found to reduce the fears of conditioned animals. (See discussion on psychopharmacological therapy in Chapter 3.)

Cognitive-behavioral therapy works by getting people to talk about and ultimately experience those things that terrify them. It also develops self-awareness and a positive attitude. This approach is believed to rewire connections and create new synapses in the brain, resulting in the formation of new memories that override old fears (Marshall,

1994). Therefore, a clinician who facilitates awareness of unconscious fears locked in the amygdala helps people to overcome their communication apprehension. The following case provides an example of the positive results of this approach.

Case Example: Fear Circuitry and Pharmacological/Cognitive-Behavioral Intervention

Lowell, an honor graduate of Princeton, suffered extreme fear about speaking in public, an integral part of his professional responsibilities as an investment analyst in a prestigious Wall Street firm. His fear was manifested in unbearable heart palpitations for which his medical doctor prescribed Inderal. Despite the alleviation of his physical symptoms from the drug, Lowell still agonized about presenting in public and enrolled in a class to overcome his fear of speaking in public. It was not until he worked through his self-defeating negative thoughts and participated in a cognitive-behavioral therapy program that included systematic desensitization of speaking fears that he overcame his communication apprehension. Lowell also eliminated his need for Inderal. He became his own beta-blocker!

Summary: Question I

The answer to the question about brain wiring seems clearly to be a resounding "yes." Evidence from research on animals and humans, tracing the fear circuitry in the brain, implicates specific cells in the amygdala and its projections and the prefrontal orbital cortex as the seat of unconscious fears that can be activated by various associations. That unconscious fears are easily evoked and that drugs and cognitive-behavioral therapy can change fear reactions are further evidence that the seat of fear lies dormant in the brain until activated. Our brains are wired in a way that predisposes humans to fear certain situations in ways that are subconscious and inaccessible. It seems quite clear that we are anatomically wired for fears through a complex fear circuitry with neurobiological and psychophysiological interactions and consequences. (See Damaisio,1995; LaDoux, 1996; Schore, 1994.)

Why Do People Fear Social Situations?

People who suffer from communication apprehension react with intense fear to situations in which there seems to be no objective source of danger. These are the times when audiences are perceived as a firing squad and interviewers as potential executioners. The real issue then becomes the source of that sense of danger that evokes such strong reactions. Where does this fear come from, and how is it differentiated from fears that emanate from reality-bound dangers such as confrontation with a wild animal or a crazed gunman? What are people really afraid of in social and performance situations?

Fear States

Fear is a phenomenon experienced by all species. It is universal. Because its manifestations are observable and measurable, it has been well studied. According to Kagan (1994), who has studied temperament in children, there are three classes of events that evoke fear states. Although related, these childhood fears are physiologically and psychologically distinct from one another (and from anxiety). The states are innate fear, conditioned fear, and fear of the unfamiliar.

Innate Fear

The first class of events that evokes fear is innate releasers—that is, instinctual reactions that produce fear states independent of experience. For example, a single experience with a preying cat can produce a state of fear in a lab rat that will last for a while and then generalize to other novel situations (Kagan, 1994). Innate fear is greater in other animals than in people. Scientists believe that innate fear has a long evolutionary history and that every vertebrate species is biologically prepared to withdraw, to attack, to become immobile, or to issue a distress call in response to a small class of events that might signal potential harm. In many animals, any pattern that resembles two staring eyes usually produces a fear state (Kagan, 1994). Kagan also demonstrated that in human infants and young children, a looming object, a loud noise, or an unexpected change in posture elicits immobility, fearful facial expressions, a sharp cry, or all three.

Case Example: Innate Fear

It is interesting that the fear of staring eyes is so common among persons suffering social phobias, especial performance anxiety. Perhaps it is the instinctive fear evoked by the staring eyes of his audience that could explain Frank's fear of speaking in public. He reported that he was not afraid of speaking, only of being looked at by an audience.

Consequently, in a class for overcoming performance anxiety, he requested opportunities to simply stand in front of the group and look back at everyone. These self-directed exercises eventually desensitized Frank's fear of visual scrutiny, a fear that many others with performance anxiety have expressed. Perhaps, like Frank, they also react to the seem-ingly reptilian stares of an audience as they would to a snake, instinc-tively sensing danger. Or might the fear of being looked at be learned?

Fear of Visual Scrutiny—Innate or Conditioned?

Although one may be conditioned to avoid visual scrutiny, with a resulting avoidance of public speaking, there is also evidence that reac-tion to eye gaze may be instinctual. Therefore, a fear of being stared at may be conditioned, innate, or a combination of both.

As mentioned in the discussion of innate releasers, fear is usually conditioned by stimuli that have the potential to create fearful response or biological reactions of uncertainty. Disapproving looks and staring eyes, just like heights and closed places, have power to destabilize a person. Flowers and puppies do not! It is not surprising that many species, including humans, fear being looked at because eye gaze is a means of threatening and establishing dominance over others. In fact, researchers can accurately predict the place of nonhu-man animals in the social hierarchy of their group by studying the eye behaviors between dominant and subordinate members (Marshall, 1994).

However, some researchers assert that eye movement is instinc-tual, hence, neurologically-based (Schore p.169–171). They point out that there are specific cells or cell clusters located in the amygdala, the anterior temporal and orbitofrontal cortices that are designed to read emotional expressions, including eye behaviors, from other persons and to implement responses (Marshall, 1994). Whatever its source, Marshall notes that ocular language is powerful and reveals a lot about relationships, running the gamut of emotions from intimacy to fury and danger. This is evidenced in the rich language for various kinds of looks, ranging from a peek to a glance to a stare to a glare to "if looks could kill." Even minute changes in gaze can influence the entire power structure of a group, determined simply by who looks at whom and how.

Perhaps the fear of being looked at is related to a feeling about one's status in a group. Hence, the fear may be instinctual (based on innate eye gaze triggers) and learned (based on cultural training about group behavior or experience in groups). Is it any wonder that like the case example of Frank, most people who fear perform-ing in public report being very uncomfortable with everyone look-ing at them when they are the center of attention? Figure 2-3a, b, c shows sketches by students in the Speaking Without Fear class who were asked to draw their fears.

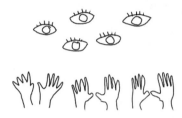

a.

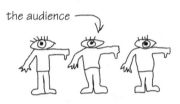

the audience

evaluation: thumbs down

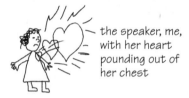

the speaker, me, with her heart pounding out of her chest

b.

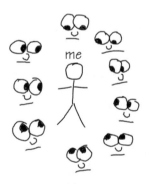

me

c.

FIGURE 2-3a-c. Illustrating fear exercise.

These line drawings are by students of a Speaking Without Fear class who visualized their fears. Staring eyes suggesting disapproval and helplessness are often themes of student drawings.

Conditioned Fear

Conditioned fear is the second class of events evoking fear. In such situations, an individual has become conditioned to enter a negative physiological state because of a repeated distinctive stimulus, such as speaking to a critical parent. Such conditioned reactions generalize to a number of associated speaking events.

Case Example: Conditioned Fear

Gina, an elegant Italian-born young woman, was a gregarious, multilingual executive who was phobic about speaking up on the job or in class, although she excelled in social situations as a hostess. She was from a traditional, patriarchal family where she learned never to question or contradict her father, who ruled his roost with an iron fist. She never understood why she was fearful of expressing her opinions in the academic or corporate worlds until she associated her adult behavior with her early conditioning by her domineering father and strict convent education, in which she learned not to question.

   This intelligent young woman ultimately found a way to leave home, requesting to attend college abroad under the guise of mastering another language, thereby circumventing one of the many cultural prohibitions to which she was subjected. However, with help in a class to overcome her seemingly inexplicable fear of speaking up and several individual therapy sessions, she became aware of the roots of her problem. She overcame her performance anxiety and nonassertiveness, especially when communicating with supervisors. Ultimately she became free enough to assert herself and express opinions and to speak in front of small and large groups. What was learned became unlearned! Released from her early programming, she changed. Gina secured a new job, moved up the corporate ladder, and improved her personal and family relationships.

Conditioned Avoidance Without Fear

Avoidance without fear can also be conditioned. A child who is not afraid of speaking in groups may "learn" to avoid speaking merely by observing a significant other do so. This behavior is clearly seen in monkeys who will avoid a snake, real or toy, if they watch another monkey display behavioral signs of fear (Kagan, 1994).

Case Example: Conditioned Avoidance of Speaking

Sarah is a prime example of conditioned avoidance of speaking. Initially convinced that she was fearful of speaking, Sarah enrolled in a class to overcome her fear. Through homework assignments and class discussions that enabled her to compare herself with others in the group, she ultimately realized that the reason she avoided speaking in a group was because her mother was petrified to do so, not because she was. She had observed her mother's behavior in various group situations and absorbed Mom's fear. However, Sarah was actually extroverted and rather enjoyed speaking up in the group once she began to participate. It was as if she came out from under a cloud and into the sunshine. She volunteered at every opportunity to question, comment, present, critique, and support others and clearly became the most outspoken person in the class.

Unfamiliar Event Fear

The third class of events producing fear is unfamiliarity. Events that are slightly different from the conscious memory of those experienced in the past provoke fear. Such discrepant events have been shown to activate the limbic system, the seat of emotional responses in the brain, which is linked to coordination of all the major brain systems—sensory, cortical, skeletal, and autonomic. Not functioning at birth, but mature enough for making comparisons at around 6 to 9 months, the limbic system accounts for the common reaction of stranger anxiety in infants of that age. By 1 year, a child shows fear to a variety of unfamiliar events, especially people. A lack of knowledge and discrepant events seems to generate fear in youngsters and, probably, in adults too.

In studies on temperament, Kagan and his collaborators (Kagan, 1994) found that the persistence of stranger anxiety and fear of novel and discrepant events are major factors in differentiating children who are at risk for becoming inhibited, fearful, and timid from extroverted youngsters. The researchers believe that inhibited children are qualitatively different from uninhibited children neurobiologically and psychophysiologically. Kagan and his associates also hypothesized that children may actually inherit inhibited temperaments that may persist through a lifetime, depending on many environmental and motivational factors. (See the discussion on individual differences in the Question 3 discussion of this chapter.)

Actually, most people rarely present or perform in public unless it is professionally required. Consequently, when called upon to do so, the task is unfamiliar, probably because most school systems provide few opportunities for students to give oral presentations.

The adult students in the classes for overcoming fear of speaking have reported rarely participating in discussion or oral presentations in elementary and high school. Many vividly recalled scrupulously avoiding making such presentations unless forced to do so, which they then endured with great trepidation or froze. These same reactions persisted while in college and professional school, as well as in the workplace. Freezing and avoidance are the most common responses of fear of the unfamiliar and are known as the fight or flight syndrome (See Chapter 4).

Unfortunately, educators at all levels seem to place more emphasis on the secondary communication skills of reading and writing, although speaking and listening skills are more frequently demanded of adults—especially managers and leaders.

Interestingly, this author (B. H.) notes that speakers and performers become increasingly more fearful with unexpected events, such as an increase in audience size (even by one or two people) or a change in a room's physical arrangement. Unfamiliarity seems to exacerbate communication apprehension, even for adults.

Case Example: Inhibited Personality and Unfamiliar Event Fear

Sam, a computer specialist born in India, was courageous and/or desperate enough to enroll in a class to overcome his fear of speaking—something he needed to do to advance professionally. He quickly realized, with some guidance, that he had always been extremely fearful as a young child and overshadowed by his outgoing older sister. This very articulate and intelligent young man was obviously suffering the effects of a lifetime of painful inhibition that was never acknowledged by his well-meaning parents. Sam had great difficulty in unfamiliar situations and speaking with strangers, not just speaking in groups, which he skillfully avoided. His avoidance of these situations reduced his immediate fright. However, it ultimately, exacerbated his fear by denying him the opportunity to gain experience in speaking in all kinds of social and professional situations. His avoidance also reinforced his fear because of the relief from tension that retreat from speaking provided.

Sam had a longer way to go than most of his classmates because of his extreme inhibition, a personality trait that affected more areas of socialization than just speaking in public. However, despite his fears, he made several successful presentations, a major triumph for Sam because he had scrupulously avoided such tasks all his life. This was a good beginning in overcoming his social anxiety, something he is determined to do with further professional help.

Chronology of Unfamiliar Event Fear

Generally, with increasing age, the fear of the unfamiliar is replaced by anxiety. Children from 3 to 5 years most commonly fear things that are discrepant and novel, such as masks and transformations of the face or body, as well as large animals and the dark. By 6 years of age children begin to anticipate harm or threat of adult evaluation, which replaces fear of a direct encounter with something unfamiliar. By adolescence, conscious fears are primarily anticipatory and involve anxiety about future relations with others, possible criticism, and school performance. Interestingly, adolescence is when social phobias usually emerge (Schneier and Welkowitz, 1996).

Why Do Fears of Speaking Occur?

What is it about speaking in front of others that so many people fear? Why are extreme reactions so universal when most individuals can socialize easily in other situations?

Evolutionary Theory of Social Anxiety

Scholars, researching fear from an evolutionary viewpoint, believe that humans and other primates have highly complex biological defense or safety systems that have evolved to protect individuals against attack. Each of these systems has several components having to do with attention, evaluation, feelings, and behaviors. Social phobia, by definition, involves fears of one's own species, in contrast to wild animal fears and phobias, which involve fear of predators. As mentioned in Chapter 1, a sense of danger arises in situations that involve making impressions on others or when people are knowingly evaluated. This is known as the self-presentation theory of social anxiety (Leary and Kowalski, 1995). Jean-Paul Sartre expressed this well when he said, "Hell is other people."[1]

Ohman (1986) hypothesized that the problem of evaluation anxiety is related to an evolutionary-based predisposition to acquire fears of social stimuli that signal dominance and aggression from others of the same species. This evolved as a by-product of the dominant hierarchies that are a common social arrangement among animals such as primates. Ohman has categorized the defense systems among humans and other primates into three levels.

Defense Levels

The first level of primate defense is nonsocial and similar to the innate, or instinctive, responses described earlier. It is marked by very rapid startle responses, hyperalertness, quick discharges of behavior, and

---

[1]Translated from *Huis-clos* [*No Exit*] *suivi de les mouches* (p. 182) by J-P Sartre, 1974, Paris: Gallimard.

movements for rapid flight. These behaviors are adaptive for escape from predators. Many researchers cited by Marshall (1994). consider phobias, panic disorder, and agoraphobia to be remnants of the early human escape adaptation.

The second level of defense that evolved among primates is the territorial system. This system regulates social organization within a species and is quite prominent in lower animals and solitary mammals. This system is characterized by display behaviors to obtain and guard a home base and attract potential mates to an animal's territory. In this way, the ability to hold, or secure, resources is established. An individual's ability to maintain his or her territories is called resource-holding potential.

According to Marshall (1994), this defense system is based on another evolutionary development, an animal's capacity to evaluate and compare the resource-holding potential of others of their species with the creature's own capabilities, to determine the others' chances of prevailing in case of conflict. The ability to evaluate and compare the competence of another with regard to oneself can save one's species. Without this ability, carnage and the eventual destruction of a species could follow because of lack of vigilance.

The third level of defense is the group living level, a subsystem that evolved from the others. This higher system, found in group-forming mammals such as humans and other primates, involves the capability to signal submissiveness, appeasement, and subservience to a more dominant individual. This necessitates hypersensitivity to signals of power and an ability to challenge or send appeasement signals, thereby permitting an individual to stay within the group rather than being driven away.

The evolution of a group living system makes it possible for individuals to live together in peace and depends on the development of a social hierarchy: a social submissive system with social fear at one end of the spectrum and social dominance at the other. Within the group, animals convey information about their strength and courage in subtle, often highly complex signs and signals. The repertoire of submissive signaling behaviors varies. In primates, it includes gaze avoidance, crouching, and fear grimacing (like an appeasing smile in humans). By appeasing the dominant animal, a weaker individual gains the opportunity to stay with the group rather than being driven out to fend alone. An animal only submitting and appeasing needs to remain highly attentive and in a state of constant physiological arousal, hypersensitive to the dominant individual in the event of a need for further submissiveness (Sagan and Druyan, 1992).

The most relevant component in this system is the role of facial expressions, especially eye movements. These serve as signs and signals that range from communicating to the dominant individual that the leaders has won, to signaling a complex emotional state of subjective feelings and physiological reactions that is collectively called fear.

Human Evolution and Social Anxiety

The scientists who have focused on the evolutionary development of social anxiety in humans hypothesize that, just as in other primate species, social anxiety has developed as part of the group living system and has become part of human genetic endowment (Marshall, 1994). In addition to the group's defensive systems noted in the section on hierarchical social arrangements, there are reassuring safety systems such as bonding, cooperative endeavors, and mutually reassuring signals that lead to and reinforce attachment between members of a social group. These socially reciprocal behaviors involve etiquette, politeness, and spontaneous expressions of affections that contribute to the coherence of the group.

When these highly evolved modes of social interaction fail to inspire a sense of safety and security or, conversely, when threat is perceived, more primitive or defensive systems come into play. Researchers believe that, possibly because of genetic influences or environmental experience, socially anxious people overemphasize and become stuck in the dominance/submissive mode and are unable to participate in the mutually reassuring safety system (Marshall, 1994).

Self-Presentational Theory

Another view of social anxiety, the self-presentational theory, looks at the circumstances in which people suffer performance fears. The situations generally involve self-presentation of status that threatens others, comparisons and self-evaluation, and the possibility of a major loss in status. Whether it is giving a speech, attending a job interview, running meetings, parties, or taking oral exams, one is jockeying for position, or risking status in a social hierarchy. People invariably compare their own strength and weakness with others and involuntarily signal submissiveness to those judged stronger than them. Not unlike competition over limited resources or display behaviors, heightened vulnerability to negative appraisal causes people to be hypervigilant and fearful.

Summary: Question 2

There are many types of fears: instinctive, conditioned, and that of the unfamiliar. The problems in social phobia and communication apprehension, in particular, seem to be made up of all of these fears. In addition, according to evolutionary theory of social anxiety, the fear is based on a primitive dread of rejection resulting in ostracism and demise. This fear is reflected in the familiar statements uttered by so many people anticipating or following a performance such as, "I'm scared to death" or "I thought I would die." However irrational it may sound at the time, fears of criticism or disapproval, of being deemed of low social worth and thus rejected, are tantamount to fears of banishment and, ultimately, death and are believed by some to be at the base of communication apprehension.

The problems underlying social fears, especially the fear of performance, are complex and generally have not been known or understood until recently. Those facing the dilemma of social fears, especially performance anxiety, usually have no understanding of the roots of their dilemma, which makes the problem even worse.

Why Are Some People More Likely to Suffer from Anxiety in General, Especially Communication Anxiety ?

From the days of Hippocrates and Galen through those of Jung, it has been noted that some people come into the world excessively restrained, wary, and cautious, with others being sociable, fearless, and even bold. Early studies were unable to fully explain the psychological variation in individuals on the basis of environmental events, childhood encounters, classical and operant conditioning, or cognitive psychology. However, comparative psychologists and behavioral biologists have long noted individual variations between members of a species or closely related strains of mice, rats, cats, dogs, wolves, pigs, cows, monkeys, and even paradise fish in their tendencies during early infancy to approach or avoid novelty (Kagan, 1994; LaDoux, 1994b). This evidence for distinctive behavioral and physiological profiles of animals early in their development suggests the influence of genetic factors in the behaviors of individual members of various species. In addition, Lorenz, the noted ethologist, also showed that each animal species inherits a preparedness to learn and behave in an adaptive way (Kagan, 1994), suggesting that children begin life with a bias that predisposes them to a particular temperament and behavior.

Temperament

Early Studies
Prompted by animal research and historic interest in the matter of temperament, two psychiatrists, Alexander Thomas and Stella Chess, began studies on the temperamental dimensions of children 40 years ago. Their

longitudinal studies focused on styles of behavior, based only on parental interviews and observations of their infants and children. Thomas and Chess (cited in Kagan, 1994), noted nine temperamental dimensions on a continuum, including general activity level, regularity, and predictability of basic functions such as hunger, sleep, elimination, initial reaction to unfamiliarity (especially approach and withdrawal), ease of adaptation to new situations, responsiveness to subtle stimulus events, amount of energy associated with activity, dominant mood (whether primarily happy or irritable), distractibility, attention span, and persistence. The researchers categorized their results into three basic categories: the easy child (known today as uninhibited), the slow to warm up child (known today as inhibited), and the difficult child. They found that only the later category of temperament persisted to adulthood because the "difficult" children were posited as more apt to have psychiatric problems.

Following those landmark studies, research on temperament was dormant for many years except for investigations into shyness in the 1970s. At that time Zimbardo and his colleagues (Zimbardo, Pilkonis, & Norwood, 1975) noted that 40% of the population described themselves as shy, and an overwhelming majority reported that they were shy, in some sense. They launched a series of investigations on shyness culminating in some of the first programs to overcome the problem. Shyness was described at that time as having four dimensions:

1. **Cognitions**: Thoughts of self-consciousness, concerns about others' views of them and negative self-evaluations.
2. **Affective States**: Shy feelings, including the awareness of anxiety and feelings of distress, nervousness, embarrassment, and awkwardness.
3. **Physiological Changes**: Included increased pulse rate, blushing, perspiration, palpitations, difficulty breathing, and "butterflies in the stomach."
4. **Behavioral Responses**: Among males diminished talking and eye contact compared to nonshy males. Among females, high frequency of head nodding and nervous smiling.

Zimbardo et al. concluded that shyness was not a natural state, but a significant psychological phenomenon that most children outgrew. Until recently, shyness has been viewed on a psychological continuum, affecting between 25% and 40% of Americans, with varying levels of intensity and disability. Today, shyness is considered a form of social anxiety, with generalized social phobia its more debilitating form. An even more extreme category of this kind of behavior is labeled an avoidant personality.

At approximately the same time as the Zimbardo
shyness, James McCrosky (1977, 1978) a Speech C
researcher and professor, brought attention to the fea
among college students and labeled the problem cc
apprehension (CA). McCrosky identified four types of C   ...ocribe
what he considered anxious reticence: trait like CA, generalized context CA, person group CA, and situation CA. He considered trait like
CA to be personality based that endured across all types of settings and
circumstances and the other types of CA the result of learning that was
cognitively based. The distinction between communication anxiety and
social anxiety is vague but most researchers in communication agreed
at that time that communication anxiety is situationally based, with
attendant physiological reactions that fluctuated according to the setting, familiarity, formality, and the degree to which the person feels
competent. McCrosky also believed that communication anxiety
became a phobia when there was a consistent reaction across circumstances regardless of mitigating circumstances.

More recently approximately 13% of the American population was
found to suffer from social phobia (Schneier and Welkowitz, 1996), that
is, having social anxiety severe enough to cause social impairment.
That means social phobia is one of the most common mental disorders.
The greatest proportion of those experiencing shyness or mild social
anxiety falls into the normal range and about 6% are considered "bor-
derline" cases that are sometimes shy, sometimes not. Age is known to
change this behavior in both directions.

Brain Chemistry

Recent findings in neuroscience have contributed to the scientific
community's interest in the work on temperament, as more has
become known about the function of the brain and its chemistry. For
example, there is evidence that the brain contains more than
150 chemicals: monoamines, amino acids, hormones, and peptides
that, along with their receptors in the brain, influence the excitability
of specific sites in the central nervous system (Kagan, 1994). The
number of combinations of these molecules exceeds 10 million. It is
obvious that individuals can inherit different concentrations of most
of these chemicals, resulting in a vulnerability to emotional states
such as sadness, depression, or anxiety. (See Chapter 3.) Therefore,
the modern theoretical definition of temperament, which refers to a
moderately stable emotional or behavioral quality appearing in childhood, now includes the influence of an inherited physiological neurochemical profile.

Recent Studies

Interested in understanding more about the relationship between brain chemistry and wiring and behavior, Kagan and his associates (Kagan, 1994; Kagan, Reznik, & Snidman, 1990) began a scientific study of temperament, using a longitudinal design on three cohorts of Caucasian children from working and middle-class homes. Equal numbers of children of both sexes who were consistently sociable, talkative, and affectively spontaneous or consistently shy, quiet, and timid were chosen. The research focused on the emotion of fear, particularly the class of fears evoked by unfamiliar events, because it involved the coordination of all the major brain systems: sensory, limbic, cortical, skeletal, and autonomic. The original longitudinal studies investigated children from 21 months through 7 years of age and included physiological profiles as well as direct, detailed behavioral observations of the children. Later studies extended the age parameters from 2 months through 13 years of age.

Two fundamental behaviors were investigated. The first was reactivity, which included ease of arousal to stimulation of age-appropriate novel and discrepant events, mostly people, that resulted in movement, crying, vocalizing, smiling, autonomic nervous system and endocrine responses, response time, intensity, and time to peak magnitude of response. The second behavior they observed was self-regulation, the quality and modulation of that quality.

Children with uninhibited temperaments at 4 months of age were observed by Kagan and associates (Kagan, 1994) to have low motor activity and minimal crying in response to unfamiliar stimuli, and were sociable and appeared to be fearless in response to discrepant events at 1 and 2 years of age. Interestingly, only one-third of these children showed low sympathetic tone (minimal increases in heart rate in response to challenge). Conversely, inhibited infants were found to have had high fetal heart rate, high heart rate at 2 months and high motor reactivity to unfamiliar stimuli at 4 months.

Kagan et al. regarded the motor reactivity in response to unfamiliar stimuli at 4 months as the primary feature of the inhibited type of infant, not only because it predicted fearful behavior, but also because it probably reflected varying thresholds of excitability in the limbic sites in the brain. A proportion of the highly reactive inhibited children also showed a large rise in heart rate in response to challenges, as well as right brain activation in their electroencephalograms (EEG), implying involvement of the nervous system, especially their brains' limbic sites. At 1 and 2 years of age these children showed signs of timidity and fearfulness in response to discrepant events.

Other physiological measurements of the inhibited group showed higher heart rates at rest, more heart rate acceleration, greater increase in pupil size, and higher levels of breakdown products of the neurotransmitter noradrenaline[2] in their urine in response to unfamiliar people and objects. In addition, higher levels of cortisol, a circulating hormone typically released in saliva in response to stress (also known as hydrocortisone), were found.

The conclusion of the Kagan et al. studies, based on group differences in peripheral physiological reactions, indicated that there was an inherited variation in the threshold of arousal in selected limbic sites that contributes to shyness in childhood and even extreme degrees of social avoidance in adults. A preservation of the initial inhibited or uninhibited behaviors, especially in those children who represented the extremes in both groups, was also found. Although some temperament changes as individuals aged were noted, Kagan and colleagues prefer to call these children "formerly" inhibited or uninhibited, because the researchers did not believe that timidity or boldness could be taught, only modified. In other words, humans enter this world with particular temperaments and distinct neurochemical profiles, based on heredity, which determine the *potential* for being inhibited or uninhibited. This implies that there has to be an environment that enables the potential behaviors to appear.

Kagan (1994) states that there can be no major changes in behavior without substantial changes in autonomic physiology. Thus, as in botany, there is a genotype, an inherited genetic profile, and a phenotype, the viable results of the interaction between the genotype and the environment. Thus, a fearful child can learn to control the urge to withdraw and, on the other hand, the environment cannot actually make a child timid. A youngster always operates in a context, and the observed behaviors and moods of each child are the products of a particular temperament reacting to specific events, just as ice, water, and steam are different forms of the same molecule exposed to different conditions. Kagan (1994) believes that there is no human quality, physical or psychological, that is free of the contribution of events within and outside of an organism. Like a pale gray fabric woven tightly of thin black horizontal threads representing biology and white vertical threads representing experience, it is impossible to detect any individual black or white threads.

---

[2]This is a chemical means of transmission across synapses in postganglionic neurons of the sympathetic nervous system and in some parts of the central nervous system, and is a precursor of epinephrine in its major biosynthetic pathway; also known as norepinephrine.

In summary, Kagan hypothesized that inhibited children belong to a qualitatively distinct category of infants who are born with a lower threshold for limbic-hypothalamic arousal to unexpected changes or novel events they cannot assimilate. These children are considered neurobiologically and psychophysiologically different, governed basically by their inherited neural chemistry and connections. However, the importance of differentiating between those who are quiet because of temperamental factors and those who have inhibition because of environmental experiences alone was recognized. Nevertheless, Kagan believes that temperamental factors contribute to the development of social anxiety, avoidance, and symptoms of panic.

Case Example: Inhibited Personality and Communication Anxiety

Examples of the obviously inhibited type personality abound in those struggling with performance anxiety. In addition to Sam, (discussed in Question 2) there is Margaret, a gentle and articulate book editor, who gave an excellent presentation on her work, which was videotaped for her to view at home. However, unlike the other students in the class on overcoming speaking fears, she adamantly refused to look at her tape. Having recalled a lifetime of painful shyness, Margaret could not bare to see herself on video. Finally, she shared with the group that her mother had been called to school by the principal when she was in second grade because she never talked in class or to anyone in school. Her timidity in groups had persisted to adulthood, when she finally felt compelled to do something about her problem because it was interfering with her professional advancement. At least she had opened a door for some change by enrolling in a class to overcome her fears about speaking in groups. Ultimately, with considerable support, she began to see herself as others saw her, as a competent, articulate spokesperson. However, she never did muster the courage to view her videotapes, although she did complete all of her speaking assignments, a major accomplishment for her. Margaret has miles to go before she overcomes her inhibited trait problems, but at least she has begun. Hopefully, she will follow up on the recommendations given to her to pursue psychotherapy and additional classes in oral presentations.

Genetic Factors in Social Anxiety

According to psychiatrist Robert Kendler (cited in Schneier & Welkowitz, 1998), who conducted a study of social phobia on 2,000 pairs of female twins, genetic inheritance accounted for about 30% of the chance of the development of social phobia. Environmental factors accounted for the remaining 70%. Other genetic studies, using different definitions of social fears, estimated that the genetic contribution varied from 22 to 50%. Hence, it was determined that some individuals may inherit a tendency toward social phobia, although in others it may be learned.

Social phobia also seems to run in families, according to research by Abby Fyer and Salvatore Mannuza (cited in Schneier & Welkowitz, 1996). They found that the rate of social phobia was three times higher in families of patients with social phobia than in families of control group subjects. However, this study's results were only for generalized social phobia and did not deal with discrete social phobia, such as that of public speaking.

Interestingly, persons with different types of social phobia have different patterns of heart rate reactions to public speaking. Persons with discrete communication anxiety note a surge in heart rate during the first minute of a performance situation, while a person with a generalized form of social phobia, even though their fear of public speaking is just as severe, show a less pronounced heart rate reaction. Hence, one group may be particularly prone to surges in physical symptoms, such as a racing heart, blushing, trembling, and sweating, especially in a performance situation, while others may have less severe physical responses, but equally or more worrisome thoughts

Brain Chemistry

Certain medications have been found to attenuate levels of social anxiety, as well as dominance and sociability in animals.

At the precursor stage, it has been hypothesized that dopamine[3] is the neurotransmitter culprit. Liebowitz believes that the low extroversion trait of social phobia sufferers might relate to their lower levels of brain dopamine (Goode, 1998). Another neurotransmitter found crucial to the brain chemistry foundation for social dominance hierarchies, the pecking order within social groups, is serotonin.[4] Animals with higher levels of serotonin have been found to be more social and dominant within the group. In addition, animals with lower levels of dominance change their behavior when treated with medications such as Prozac, which increases levels of serotonin (Raleigh et al, 1991).

These results corroborate findings that differences in brain chemistries predispose some people to social anxiety, hence performance anxiety.

---

[3]This is a form of dopa and occurs as a neurotransmitter in the brain and as an intermediate in the biosynthesis of epinephrine.

[4]A powerful vasoconstrictor found especially in the brain, blood serum, and gastric mucous membrane.

Personality Influences

Suggestibility and Self-Deception

Dr. Ian Wickramasekera, a physiological psychologist, has presented evidence of the contribution of certain personality traits to the development of somatization and psychophysiological disease (Wickramasekera, 1998). He has developed a high-risk model of threat perception (HRMTP). The model postulates that people who score high or low on tests of absorption (absorption, or suggestibility, related to the ability to be hypnotized) and/or score high on the Marlowe-Crown scale have a high likelihood of somatization and psychophysiological disease. The Marlowe-Crown scale measures a person's capacity to repress or block aversive perceptions, memories, and moods from consciousness, a process that appears to operate by promoting inattention to aversive situations and by amplifying positive situations (Crown & Marlowe, 1960). People with severe performance anxiety are considered by this author (B. H.) to suffer the effects of somatization because their mental perceptions of danger result in intense physiological reactions.

According of Wickramasekera (personal communication, 1999) highly suggestible people are very empathic and often hypersensitive, tending to see in or read into a situation things that are not there. Consequently, they may have poor ego boundaries and easily suffer the fears and pain of others. Conversely, those who are not very suggestible are hyposensitive, not in touch with their physiological responses and/or feelings and are less able to deal with psychological phenomena, in which they do not generally believe (Wickramasekera, personal communication, 1999). However, the bodies of these persons know what their mind does not acknowledge and react without the individual's awareness. Those with low suggestibility need to be shown (with biofeedback instrumentation), rather than told, about the mind-body connection. People high in self-deception, whose suppression of affect can block things out of their consciousness, may feel the stress physiologically, but not recognize or realize it because of their limitations (Wickramasekera, 1998).

The HRMPT model for psychophysiological dysfunction has potential for identifying personality traits that contribute and or exacerbate performance anxiety, thereby suggesting additional ways of treating such individuals. Note the following case of Jill, someone high in absorption, which illustrates its effects on her behavior.

Case Example: High Suggestibility and Communication Apprehension

Jill, a very animated and articulate executive, reported that she never had any problem with public speaking until she was on a panel with a colleague who was so terrified that she could hardly get through her presentation. Since that experience, Jill had extreme fears of speaking in groups, an integral part of her job. She even said that she could barely listen to and watch classmates give presentations, because she knew that they were apprehensive. She lived (perhaps died would be more accurate) with each presenter. Jill was an example of someone with surplus empathy and poor ego boundaries, who identified so much with the performance anxiety of others that she became frightened of speaking in groups, something she had never before feared. Once she understood the reasons for her hyperarousal, she overcame her problem, finally saying, "What's the big deal?" (See also case example of Sarah in the "**Conditioned**" section in this chapter.)

Perfectionism

People who show tendencies toward perfectionism and excessive need of approval or control also have been found to be prone to anxiety disorders and are highly anxious about performing in public (Bourne, 1995, p. 226–228). One slip, a change of a word or planned action, an unanticipated question, or a disapproving frown (perceived or real) is enough to throw people with these characteristics into a tizzy. They often blame their excessive arousal on a *faux pas* in their planning or delivery: something rarely, if ever, observable to their audience.

An inordinate and inappropriate need for perfectionism, approval, or control usually originates in early childhood experiences. Either it is learned directly from significant others or the demands for perfectionism and achievement are observed and internalized. Conversely, these traits can develop as a response to criticism endured during childhood. Hence, as adults, perfectionists strive to do everything perfectly, constantly seeking reassurance and approval.

Examples of perfectionist reactions abound and lurk just beneath the surface in many students who are terrified to present to a group lest they fail or disappoint themselves or others. This is often the case even with novice performers with no experience, who talk freely about their feelings when questioned. Ultimately perfectionists can learn to recognize the negative effects of their perfectionism and work to reduce their self-defeating unrealistic standards. Perfectionists have to realize that the real enemy is within. As in a paraphrase of cartoonist Walt Kelly's famous Pogo quote[5]: I have met the enemy, and he is I.

---

[5]"I have met the enemy and he is us."

Cognitive Dissonance

Another type of problem has been found by the author (B.H.) to be a basis of communication apprehension with some individuals—that of cognitive dissonance. This problem is a mental conflict, often unconscious, that occurs when people feel compelled to violate certain of their core values, beliefs, or attitudes. It can surface when individuals live under an oppressive political system or work for organizations whose values conflict with their own. Indecision or avoidance can be manifestations of cognitive dissonance.

Case Examples: Cognitive Dissonance

James, an experienced electrical engineer, who later opted for a career on Wall Street analyzing stocks, personifies a communicative anxiety based on a conflict of core values (cognitive dissonance). A competent engineer and ethical person, James was very uncomfortable promoting companies he did not believe were solid, but had no problems giving presentations on objective engineering topics. He did not understand the source of his communication apprehension until he became aware of his deep conflict about promoting flimsy stocks, unfortunately an integral part of James's commission-based job.

David, a frustrated Israeli history scholar wanted to teach, but was unhappily trapped in a lucrative family business selling furniture. His job entailed presentations to groups of buyers, something he found very difficult to do. He did not understand his performance anxiety until he made a seamlessly assured presentation on his passion, the history of the Middle East, in the class he enrolled in to overcome his fear of speaking. Finally realizing the source of his dilemma, David planned to leave the family business and with it his performance anxiety, to pursue his first love, teaching history.

Other examples of the effects of cognitive dissonance on performance have been observed in many persons who grew up in Communist Bloc or totalitarian regimes. Warned by their parents never to talk to anyone about their family's beliefs or values for fear of serious reprisals on the family, many fortunate enough to emigrate to the United States harbored these childhood admonitions until adulthood with no awareness of their buried memories or conflicts. The following case exemplifies this kind of problem.

Graciela, a Cuban-born school psychologist, dropped out of her doctoral program because of her fear of oral presentations and oral examinations. She also suffered greatly when she had to testify in court representing abused children. Graciela never understood her inordinate fear about speaking until she began to talk about her early years growing up in Cuba as a child of capitalist parents who had owned land and a factory before the revolution on the island. Her parents had warned her never to speak to anyone outside of her family, especially about family matters. Only after she recognized the source of her unconscious conflict, to speak or not to speak, was she able to do so without panic. Free at last, she returned to her doctoral program. Her insights and relief came through assignments and discussions in the class of Speaking Without Fear, which she had enrolled in to overcome her fear that had seriously interfered with her professional progress in her adopted country.

Summary: Question 3

All people have unique inherited dispositions based on their neurobiology and psychophysiology that contribute to individual variations in their response to fear. These differences affect their thoughts, feelings, and behavior. Some individuals may be hypersensitive to social signals and overreact to ambiguous signals, such as body language. Others may interpret social signals normally, but have an overactive chemical response to stressors that leads to adrenaline being pumped into the bloodstream at the slightest hint of a threat or easily activates certain body organs such as muscles, the heart, or sweat glands. Still others may be acutely sensitive to what is going on inside their bodies and respond to that, creating even more intense mental fears. However, the environment influences the chemistry of the brain as much as the brain influences the way a person interacts with the world. Biological tendencies interact with life experiences to shape what people become.

What Role Does Learning and Perception Play in Social Phobia/Performance Anxiety?

> There is nothing either good or bad, but thinking makes it so—*Hamlet*, Act 2, Scene 2—William Shakespeare[6]

Not all fears are instinctive and not all people have highly reactive nervous systems. Why then are so many people fearful of performing in public, even when they are trained, skilled, and prepared to do so? To address this issue, it is necessary to discuss behavioral theories, especially the types of conditioning and thoughts that are related to irrational fears.

[6]From *The Annotated Shakespeare* (p. 218), edited by A. L. Rowse, 1978, New York: Orbis.

Behavioral Theories

Classical Conditioning

Scientific thinking in the 1920s (Milhollan & Forisha, 1972) attributed all behavior to classical conditioning, more commonly known as stimulus-response theory. That is, if you pair a loud, frightening siren with a neutral object such as a white, furry bunny, a child should develop a fear of the rabbit and also of all white furry objects.

The same pairing can occur with social fears. Once an emotionally charged experience and a previously neutral situation are paired, they become powerfully linked in a person's mind. These fears are easy to acquire, but difficult to shed. This author (B.H.) has worked with many people with a discrete anxiety of performance whose fears about communicating seemed clearly classically conditioned. They were people who recalled one traumatic event that had triggered their fear of speaking (recall the examples of Nancy and George cited earlier.) Their experiences invariably involved humiliation, such as being laughed at or embarrassed in a social or school situation.

Operant Conditioning

A variation of the classical conditioning theory is operant conditioning, which explains fears as the culmination of a long series of small negative experiences and consequences rather than a response to a single traumatic event. B. F. Skinner, a psychologist, refined the principles of operant conditioning by teaching pigeons to play ping pong with the use of rewards to encourage a particular behavior, which he called learning (Milhollan & Forisha, 1972).

Skinner believed that all behaviors, including fearful responses, were shaped in predictable ways by the past experiences of consequences that followed particular behaviors (Milhollan & Forisha, 1972). For example, a rat will avoid the part of the cage in which it receives a shock and visit the part of the cage where food is dispensed. The rat's behavior was shaped by the consequences of being in certain locations of the cage.

Humans respond to operant conditioning in a similar fashion. If one grows up with praise and reward from significant others for certain social behaviors such as speaking up or expressing opinions, the individual is more likely to do so as an adult. Conversely, if there is frequent criticism (a punishing consequence) for speaking up or giving controversial opinions, one is more likely to develop fear and shy away from situations requiring speaking up as an adult. A young girl whose singing is repeatedly ignored or mocked is less likely to feel confident about her ability to perform vocally years later. Such was the case with Barbra Streisand, who suffered serious stage fright for many years despite her acclaim and success (Schneier and Welkowitz, 1996), as well as with Gina, the elegant Italian executive cited in an earlier case example.

However, those suffering the debilitating consequences of negative conditioning do not generally understand the effects of any type of conditioning on behavior. People tend to attribute their fears to an event or feeling that occurred just prior to their fear reaction. They are more apt to say, "I cut my speech short because I was nervous," rather than, "I cut my speech short because I have a history of my anxiety being relieved when I stop speaking." It would not have been the immediate or preceding event or feeling that shaped behavior in such a case, but rather the relief (escape) that influenced the behavior.

Classical conditioning models ask a socially anxious person to recall the early traumatic events that triggered social fear and avoidance, with the operant model asking what consequences, positive or negative, were experienced when entering and leaving the fearful social situations. Both models emphasize the influence of specific problem behavior in a person's life, rather than the influence of complex emotional experiences such as fear and anxiety.

Cognitive Theory

Cognitive psychologists who believe that to understand people, thoughts and feelings require attention, have challenged the simple classical and operant conditioning models. They believe it is not merely a question of stimulus, response, or consequence, for all the praise in the world will not erase a social fear if the fearful person rejects praise and clings to irrational fears or embarrassment. Understanding the negative thoughts accompanying anxiety provides a new path to explain and manage social fears.

> Suppose they find out I'm scared . . . what if I forget what I'm going to say . . . they will think I'm a fool . . . a phony. . . . they will see me trembling . . . know I'm a nervous wreck . . . what are they thinking of me?

Any of these thoughts are enough to fuel the stress response and generate an instantaneous neurochemical cascade initiated in the amygdala and cortex (see Chapters 3 and 4), creating physiological symptoms that divert attention from a task at hand, such as delivering a message or a toast at a wedding.

The cognitive model considers how thoughts influence feelings and behavior. It posits that dwelling on negative thoughts, which are generally irrational or untrue, causes negative emotional responses that effect harmful changes in behavior. These behavioral changes from negative thoughts, in turn, cause people to think that they have nothing to say or that they will be "found out." Some people react by having complete pessimism about how they will do in certain situations. In contrast, confident speakers may occasionally have such thoughts, but rise to the occasion as needed.

Negative thought preoccupation is toxic, resulting in increased fear of a situation that is not dangerous. Negative thoughts are often triggered by certain events or situations such as appearing before an audience and expecting a punishing consequence. However, the punishment is usually self-inflicted by the fearful speaker, not the audience

The problem is in the thinking, not simply that people are inadequate or incompetent. Socially fearful people have been found to think differently from others. They have more negative thoughts about their performance, compared to subjects with general anxiety and those without anxiety, and consistently underestimate the quality of their performance (Schneier and Welkowitz, 1996). People who always feel badly about their performance deny themselves the positive reinforcement that naturally follows a satisfactory performance, thereby interfering with the development of self-confidence.

Fearful thoughts also tend to build on one another. What may start as a fleeting, negative thought may increase until there is a cascade of catastrophic thoughts and helpless feelings. Albert Ellis, the originator of cognitive therapy, argues that most emotional problems are linked to core categories of negative thoughts or presumption (Ellis, 1962). First, if one thinks that he or she must be perfect or loved by everyone, the individual is bound to feel like a failure because such a state is impossible. Further, when people believe they "must" or "should" do or be something, they set themselves up for disappointment and emotional pain.

However, just as pure classical conditioning or operant behavioral theory has limitations, so does purely cognitive theory. Experience, alone, does not seem to correct distorted thinking. That is, even when people succeed in performing in feared social situations, such as giving an oral presentation, it is hard for them to interpret and accept the success. As Shakespeare's Hamlet implied, you are, after all, what you think.

As noted previously, fears are hard to extinguish. Therefore, in recent years behavioral and cognitive approaches to social fears have been combined to help individuals with social phobia. This approach defines and seeks to remediate both thought and behavior. Avoidance, which develops as a result of fears, is dealt with in concert with the fears, themselves, which are recognized and discussed. The combination of approaches leads to greater awareness and creates positive experiences that are effective in overcoming social phobias, including communication apprehension, even for timid individuals.

Perception

One other concept intertwined with negative thinking and learning is perception, a complex phenomenon touching on other issues in communication anxiety. It is easy to understand that "beauty is in the eye of the beholder" or that "love is blind," because it is what people perceive and believe that causes particular ways of behaving. People's behavior is based on their perception of themselves: that is, their self-concept or self-image.

Self-concept is actually a collection of an individual's self-perceptions. This includes such views of the self as physical appearance, mental capacity, life roles, skills, achievements, and ability to perform. Self-concept is a product of many influences, primarily stemming from the early years, but in the present, as well. These influences include how people considered important to one react to a person (looking-glass view), comparisons of oneself with others (self-comparison view), and the roles (e.g., family, community, professional) one plays in life (role view).

Self-concept also acts as a filter of others' statements about individuals. If one doesn't think that he or she does something well, the person automatically looks for and listens to statements that reinforce the negative self-perception. If complimented, a person with a poor self-concept will generally disregard, discount, or rationalize the compliment. Very often, the problems of speaking in public can be traced to a low self-image rather than to any external factors or to an inability to express oneself. People who feel positively about themselves may reflect confidence and have little difficulty in a wide variety of situations, because self-concept influences interpretations of language and events. Even though some people with a positive self-concept may experience communication anxiety for a host of other reasons, the more positive their self-concept, the more likely they will be to expect and accept success.

Distorted Self-Perceptions

Many speakers have no idea about how they are seen by others. Fearful speakers are usually convinced that any nervousness is apparent for all to see and that their performance is inadequate. Even when they have positive feedback, it is often disregarded.

Or, they may not be themselves in front of a group and attempt to impress, rather than express. This creates a feeling of restraint, as if they are playing an uncomfortable role, causing them to be so concerned about the trappings of a presentation that they have difficulty focusing on the message.

Johari Window

Drs. Joe Luft and Harry Ingham (Luft, 1970) developed the Johari Window (Figure 2-4), a useful tool for visualizing a person's many selves. The quadrants, to be considered as panes in a window, work to illustrate a person's public and private self. The model helps people realize that their self-perceptions are often inaccurate. The upper-left quadrant, open, or public self, represents the known self that one is willing to share with others. The size of the quadrant for a particular individual depends on the amount of trust existing in a relationship or situation. The lower-left quadrant, hidden, or private, represents the known self that one cannot share with others. The upper-right quadrant, blind, represents the part of a person that is unknown to oneself and known to others. The lower-right quadrant, unknown, represents the part that is not known to oneself or to others.

The size of each quadrant is flexible and will change according to a person's feelings, relationships with others, the situation, and the individual's level of self-knowledge. As communicators and performers gain information about themselves through feedback from others, as well as from viewing videotapes of their performances, their hidden and blind selves are reduced. Corrections of distorted self-perceptions help performers/communicators reduce their fears and become more comfortable in front of an audience.

THE JOHARI WINDOW

	Known to Self	Unknown to Self
Known to Others	Open/Public Self	Blind Self
Unknown to Others	Hidden/Private Self	Unknown Self

FIGURE 2-4. The Johari window.

Case Example: Blind Self

Forrest, a computer specialist with no experience giving presentations in public, had very unrealistic expectations and little awareness about his speaking ability. He believed that he could speak to any group with the same aplomb and charisma as his father, a prominent minister. Because he was blind about how he came across to others, he winged his presentations. However, he changed quickly when his blind self was reduced with the help of feedback from classmates and his own reactions to himself on videotape. It helped him realize the necessity for appropriate preparation and to be himself, not his father!

Summary: Question 4

Whatever the innate disposition of a person, early conditioning and social learning has a major influence on the development of self-concept. A negative self-concept can be the foundation for some cases of communication anxiety. However, equally important are thought patterns, because negative thinking and unrealistic perceptions of oneself create irrational thinking that can also precipitate and perpetuate social and performance anxiety.

What Role Does Culture Play in the Etiology of Communication and Performance Anxiety?

Every society is governed by codes of thinking, customs, and behavior that are culturally determined. These codes determine how and to whom one speaks and are based on gender, age, and status. They include nonverbal behaviors such as posture, eye contact, facial expressions, tone of voice, posture, rules of proximity, degrees of self-disclosure, and displays of emotion.

Cultural rules are neither obvious nor spoken, and learning them is like learning a language. Children acquire them, usually without questioning. As adults, unspoken cultural rules become hooks that unconsciously govern the way people behave. Cultural hooks are particularly troublesome for people who need or wish to adapt to another culture, either because they emigrate or wish to become assimilated in an adopted country. This may also be the case when people move up the socioeconomic ladder and socialize in different circles or move to different regions within the same culture (rural to urban).

Although there are differences in the ways that other anxieties are manifested across societies, social and performance anxiety are similar in every culture (Barlow, 1998). Such symptoms as blushing and accelerated heart rate appear among aborigines as well as New Yorkers, depending on a person's unique physiology and heredity, which both contribute to the manifestation of specific symptoms. Nevertheless, in every culture, life experiences and backgrounds have a major impact on social anxiety, especially communication and performance anxiety.

The expression of feelings, in particular, is well known to be culturally determined. The intensity of emotion expressed by Southern European and Mediterranean cultures, compared to Northern European cultures is as legendary as the inhibition of emotions by certain Eastern cultures. When there are crossovers in cultures, unconscious problems about communicating in public often arise.

As with ethnic groupings, organizations have cultures with rules of behavior that can be problematic for people who do not understand or adjust to them. Communication anxiety problems inherent in cross-cultural differences and conflicts within families and organizations are explored in the following material.

Generational Conflicts

When children of immigrants or first-generation (or longer) Americans are exposed to one set of cultural rules at home and another in the school and community, conflicts may occur. These conflicts can affect attitudes about performance. Speakers of any age can experience considerable anxiety when presenting a speech, if they have been steeped in a cultural tradition that frowns on assertiveness, emotional displays, or being the center of attention. Participating in events that include or demand these behaviors can feel rude or abrasive to some people from Eastern cultures with display rules in which public behavior is expected to be polite, even humble. Such expectations vary dramatically from Western behaviors.

Case Examples: Cultural Dilemmas

Mei, an articulate, highly educated Korean-American archivist, thought she would faint when first asked to comment from her seat in a class that she enrolled in to overcome her overwhelming fear of speaking. Gradually, through discussion and reflection as a result of some homework assignments, it became clear that the root of her fears was a conflict of cultural rules, a thought that had never occurred to her. As a child Mei had been taught to value humility, politeness, even stoicism, and was never allowed to display her feelings in public. Speaking up was not considered a virtue in her Korean background, although it was an asset in the American culture, especially in her profession. She had managed to complete college and graduate school in the United States without giving an oral presentation and was a master at avoiding such assignments on her job. Yet, Mei's career advancement depended on her ability to speak in public, and she was panic-stricken. However, once she understood the source of her conflict and gained some experience and positive feedback from her audience, she lost her fear and became a superb speaker. Her personal transformation was rapid and dramatic!

Noriko, a soft-spoken and gentle Japanese-American architect, was a clear example of a Japanese-American cross-cultural dilemma that caused untoward communication apprehension. Noriko had to present and defend her design plans to a jury as part of her apprenticeship in a prestigious architectural firm. However, when all eyes were on her, she was so anxious she could hardly speak. Noriko actually admitted feeling "abrasive and aggressive" when she was the center of attention, a place completely antithetical to her traditional cultural background. This was far from the case, according to her audience, who viewed her as charming, informative, and interesting.

Noriko, like Mei, never realized the depth of her cultural conflict. Although she was born in the United States, her upbringing was sufficiently Japanese for her to incorporate the message that no Japanese woman should speak her mind, especially in public, or show emotions such as enthusiasm, even though her profession required her to do so. Despite her lifetime in the United States and her prestigious Ivy League education, Noriko did not understand or accept Western cultural attitudes and genuinely believed that assertiveness was impolite. Perhaps in Japan, a soft-spoken voice and lowering of the eyes is considered a virtue, but in the United States it is not. With awareness of her cultural conflicts, along with support and encouragement to embrace American cultural rules, Noriko's communication apprehension diminished.

The cases of Mei and Noriko reflect the varying views about reticence between Eastern and Western cultures. Westerners see shyness as a sign of personal weakness, but in other cultures, even among Hindus in India, it is customary and a sign of respect to lower the eyes, especially in the presence of culturally defined superiors. It is no wonder that many students from these backgrounds, both men and women, struggle with cultural conflicts about assertiveness and communication that have significant professional and personal consequences in the West.

Gender and Cultural Dilemmas

According to Schneier and Welkowitz (1996), twice as many women as men struggle with social anxiety, possibly because of hormonal differences. The investigators believe that because women are more dependent on relationships, loss of approval and social demands are especially important to them. However, in the United States, more men than women were found to seek treatment for social anxiety. Schneier and Welkowitz say that the predominance of men seeking help for social anxiety relates to the cultural expectations of male aggressiveness that continues in our society. For men to advance in most management careers or become leaders in any endeavor, they are expected to have good oral communication skills, especially public speaking and conducting meetings. Therefore, males feel especially vulnerable when they are anxious about presenting in front of a group (Schneier and Welkowitz, 1996).

However, of approximately 800 students enrolled in classes of Speaking Without Fear taught by this author (B. H.), there has been an equal distribution of men and women. It seems that with more professional opportunities open to women today, they face the same dilemmas as men. Perhaps this is because assertiveness, an attribute that some women lack depending on their cultural backgrounds, temperament, experience, and training, is basic to leadership. Furthermore, women are expected to be as good as men and yet maintain their femininity, a difficult role to play for many female managers and executives. Hence, the progress that has been made in creating more opportunities for women is a double-edged sword and can account for the influx of women in courses offering help for communication anxiety.

Case Example: Assertiveness Problem

Doris, a seemingly flighty administrative assistant, was very loquacious, except with her boss, whom she viewed as abusive. She was terrified of speaking to him about anything important and was convinced that she was inept and a failure. Once she became aware of how her nonassertiveness with him reinforced her boss' offensive behavior toward her and learned some assertive strategies, Doris' attitudes and, ultimately, her behavior changed. She began to cope with her boss, as well as with others who intimidated, her in an assertive manner (not aggressive or nonassertive) and reduced her fears about speaking to authorities. Doris also learned how others viewed her and curtailed her nervous mannerisms, which were perceived by others as flightiness.

Summary: Question 5

Unconscious cultural conflicts underlie many cases of communicative performance anxiety, especially with persons from non-Western backgrounds. Gender problems and role conflicts in organizations also create serious problems, especially for women who have traditionally been raised to be nonconfrontational and feminine, even in the West. Nonassertiveness and communication anxiety interfere with the leadership opportunities open to today's women, who must compete in what may still be a man's world.

Other Factors that Precipitate and/or Perpetuate Communication Anxiety

People who suffer from communicative performance anxiety struggle with many common misperceptions and negative thoughts about performance that either precipitate or perpetuate their anxiety. Many of these issues probably result from the secrecy that surrounds the problem, which is generally not discussed or understood, even in professional or educational circles. In general, there seems to be a lack of knowledge or misunderstanding about the following facts.

Prevalence

Most people who suffer communication apprehension do not realize the prevalence of the problem and believe that they are unique, weak, or sick. Therefore, they avoid performance situations completely. However, avoidance achieves only temporary relief. The long-range effects of avoidance, a self-defeating coping style, are to reinforce the fear.

Normal Arousal Versus Negative Anxiety

Many people with communication anxiety misunderstand the source of their apprehension. A certain amount of arousal is normal for any challenge, such as speaking at an important event or before an audience, and is not all bad. Known as eustress (good stress), it involves a state of physiological arousal that can be channeled and useful, if understood and not feared. That physiological state can be likened to that of a race horse at the starting gate, all charged up and ready to go, or to the emotions and reactions of an athlete before a big event. The physiological arousal that occurs in the body in a moment of challenge keeps a person alert and energized. However, if eustress is viewed as abnormal or misconstrued as unnatural or undesirable, it can easily escalate to a state of distress that interferes with optimal performance.

The distinction between physiological arousal and subjective anxiety is important. Physiological arousal is the body's natural, adaptive response to a challenge that cannot and should not be completely eliminated. (See Chapter 4.) Subjective anxiety is the negative interpretation of an event or person perceived as threatening or dangerous. That distinction must be clearly understood for individuals to gain control over inordinate fears about communicating. If understood, natural physiological arousal to a challenge can be productively channeled to enhance all types of performance. (See Chapter 4.)

Stress Misconceptions

Stress begins in the mind because it is based on an individual's appraisal of an event. That appraisal is related to the person's values, beliefs, experiences, and coping resources. Attitudes about stressful events evolve in a social context and are based on an individual's sense of acceptance or rejection in social interactions. Each individual has unique stressors (or triggers), people, or events, that set off their stress response, a physiological phenomenon related to conscious attitudes or unconscious memories that evoke fear. One person's stress can be another's challenge.

Communication Misconceptions

Many people who have problems with interviews and giving speeches have no concept of what communication is really about. More that just unidirectional talking, communicating is an ongoing, dynamic, mutually reciprocal, and influential process that involves verbal and nonverbal messages. Whether it is one to one, as in an interview, or takes place in a small or large group, communication involves analysis of the audience, listening, interpretation, and feedback. Good speakers are good communicators who prepare purposeful messages carefully and, like an agile prizefighter, are capable of adjusting, proactively and reactively, to feedback.

Semantic Interpretations

Words have the power to create undue pressure on speakers. Note the different reactions evoked by the following expressions and synonyms and how they vary based on feelings and perceptions.

Negative	Neutral or Positive
Giving a speech	Communicating a message
Speech	Enlarged conversation
Nervousness	Physiological arousal
Dread	Challenge
Fail	Succeed
Audience/Judges	Listeners/conversational partners
Cannot	Can
Avoid	Cope/manage
Impress	Express
Try	Do

Attitudes about performance can be changed by being aware of the power of the words used to describe feelings and events.

Lack of Preparation

Effective oral presentations require knowledge about how to prepare various types of messages. Most work on a presentation is done behind the scenes and entails thoughtful planning and preparation. Delivery of any message, like the icing on the cake, cannot substitute for poor ingredients or content. Being unprepared is an invitation for failure.

Lack of Rehearsal and Inexperience

Novice presenters are often plagued by unrealistic expectations and therefore are disappointed with their first attempts to speak in public. Realistic expectations, coupled with adequate preparation, rehearsals, and, ultimately, experience are as essential for speakers and performers in the arts as they are for athletes and musicians. However, in an effort to compensate for their communication anxiety, many people over- or underprepare, thereby creating more, rather than less, tension. Although preparation is essential, overdoing may leave no room for spontaneity, although inadequate or inappropriate preparation is also a major problem for obvious reasons.

Being Yourself

People often are unwilling or unable to be themselves and get caught up in trying to impress instead of express. It is better to be oneself, the most effective self possible, rather than to attempt to be someone you are not or to emulate someone else. Useful maxims are "Express, don't impress" and "Be yourself—your best self."

Misperceptions

Most people with communicative performance anxiety are convinced that their nervousness is very apparent, which is generally not the case. Accelerated heart rates, trembling muscles, even an omission or last-minute switch in presenting planned ideas are generally not noticeable to an audience. Secondly, people frequently misperceive what the audience is thinking and engage in a kind of mind reading. Such speakers are convinced that their audience has a very negative opinion of their performance, when the reverse is frequently the case. Finally, speakers often perceive only the negative aspects of their performance, thereby distorting reality and precluding positive feedback.

Distorted Thinking

There are a host of other distorted thought processes, such as overgeneralizations (once bad, always bad), polarized thinking (all or none), and catastrophizing (I'm going to fail), which play havoc with speakers' perceptions of themselves and their presentation. Such distorted thoughts must be identified and refuted.

Understanding the Speech Motor Processes

Some people focus on words rather than ideas when speaking, which causes considerable anxiety. This is because they do not understand the complex process of speaking that begins as an idea in the mind. Thoughts are then encoded into language and, ultimately, into words and sentences, not the reverse. Focusing on ideas is often sufficient to generate the words and sentences necessary to express ideas. This is similar to the working of a computer software program, where ideas are the icons software that select and direct the output (communication).

Additional Overview

People with performance anxiety must recognize that they are not unique or alone, because the problem is prevalent and universal. They must also understand the interactive nature of communication, which is a dynamic process. It is equally important to understand the transpersonal nature of stress, which involves perceptions of acceptance or rejection in a social context, which can set off a stress response, the body's adaptive response to fear. Presenters must also accept that arousal to a challenge is normal and that effective performance of all types demands knowledge of message preparation, delivery, and rehearsal. They must also understand the process of how thoughts are encoded into language in order to avoid focusing on words alone when speaking. Finally, they must dispel many of their misperceptions about themselves and their distorted thoughts and recognize the power that language has on thinking, feeling, and, ultimately, performance.

Chapter Summary

Communication apprehension/performance anxiety is a complex phenomenon with common symptoms but various etiologies that involve predisposing, precipitating, and perpetuating factors. These factors include neurobiological, psychophysiological, environmental (learned), cultural, cognitive, temperament, and personality traits. In addition, naïveté, as well as ignorance about the nature of social anxiety, and the act of communication performance, itself, contributes to the problem of communication apprehension.

References

Andreassi, J. (2000). *Psychophysiology: Human behavior and physiological response*. Hillsdale, NJ: Laurence Erlbaum.

Barlow, D. H. (1988). *Anxiety and its disorders*. New York: Guilford Press.

Beck, A. (1979). *Cognitive therapy and emotional disorders*. New York: American Library.

Benson, H. (1975). *The relaxation response*. New York: Avon Books.

Bourne, E. J. (1995). The Anxiety & Phobia Workbook, Oakland, CA: New Harbinger Publications Inc. p. 226–228.

Browne T. & Bhat, N. (1997). *Anger and hostility control using heart rate variability biofeedback*. Short course presented at the Association for Applied Psychophysiology and Biofeedback meeting, San Diego.

Carson, R. (1983). *Taming your gremlin*. New York: Harper Perennial.

Crown, D. P. & Marlowe, D. (1960). A new scale of social desirability independent of psychopathology. *Journal of Consulting Psychology, 24,* 349–354.

Damasio, A. R. (1994). *Descartes' error: Emotion, reason and the human brain*. New York: Putnam.

Davis, M. (1992). The role of the amygdala in conditioned fear. In J. P. Aggleton (Ed.), *The amygdala: Neurobiological aspects of emotion, memory, and mental functions*. New York: Wiley-Liss.

Ellis, A. (1962). *Reason and emotion in psychotherapy*. New York: Lyle Stuart.

Everly, G. & Rosenfeld, R. (1981) *The nature and treatment of the stress response: A practical guide for clinicians*. New York: Plenum Press.

Fried, R. (1987). Relaxation with biofeedback-assisted guided imagery: The importance of breathing rate as an index of hypoarousal. *Biofeedback and Self-Regulation, 12,* 273–278.

Glisky M., Tataryn D., Tobias, B., Kihlstrom J., & McConkey, K. (1991). Absorption, openness to experience and hypnotizability. *Journal of Personality and Social Psychology, 60,* 263–272.

Goleman, D. (1995). *Emotional intelligence*. New York: Bantam Books.

Goode, E. (1998, October 29). Old as society: Social anxiety is yielding secrets. *New York Times*. pp. 10, 12.

Grey, B. B. & England, G. (Eds.). (1969). Stuttering and the conditioning therapies. *Proceedings of the International Seminar in Stuttering and Behavior Therapies, 1966*. Monterey, CA: Monterey Institute for Speech and Hearing.

Hall, S. (1999, February 28). The anatomy of fear. *New York Times Magazine*, Section 6, p. 79.

Handly, R. & Neff, P. (1985). *Anxiety and panic attacks: Their cause and cure.* New York: Fawcett Crest.

Heimberg, R., Liebowitz, M., Hope, D., & Schneier, F. (1995). *Social phobia: Diagnosis, assessment, and treatment.* New York: Guilford Press.

Kagan, J. (1994). *Galen's prophecy: Temperament in human nature.* New York: Basic Books.

Kagan, J., Reznik, J. S., & Snidman, N. (1987). Temperamental variation in response to the unfamiliar. In N. A. Krasnegor, E. M. Blass, M. A. Hofer, & W. P. Smotherman (Eds.), *Perinatal development: A psychobiological perspective* (pp. 421–440). Orlando, FL: Academic Press.

Kagan, J., Reznik, J. S., & Snidman, N. (1990). The temperamental qualities of inhibition and lack of inhibition. In M. Lewis & S. M. Miller (Eds.), *Handbook of developmental psychopathology* (pp. 219–226). New York: Plenum Press.

Kaplan, H. (Ed.). (1996). *Psychosocial stress: Perspectives on structure, theory, life course, and methods.* New York: Academic Press.

Kapp, B. S., Pascoe, J. P., & Bixler, M. A. (1984). The amygdala: A neuroanatomical systems approach to its contributions to aversive conditioning. In L. R. Squire & N. Butters (Eds.), *Neuropsychology of Memory.* New York: Guilford Press.

Kihlstrom, J. (1984). Cognitive unconscious. *Science, 48,* 1445–1452.

LaDoux, J. E. (1994a). The amygdala: Contributions to fear and stress. *Seminars in the Neurosciences, 6,* 231–237.

LaDoux, J. E. (1994b, June). Emotion, memory, and the brain. *Scientific American, 270,* 50–57.

LaDoux, J. E. (1996). *The emotional brain.* New York: Simon & Schuster.

Leary, M. & Kowalski, R. (1995). *Social anxiety.* New York: Guilford Press.

Luft J. (1970). *Group processes: An introduction to group dynamics.* Palo Alto, CA: National Press Books.

Marshall, J. (1994). *Social phobia: From shyness to stage fright.* New York: Basic Books.

McCrosky, J. C. (1970). Measures of communication-bound anxiety. *Speech Monographs, 37,* 269–277.

McCrosky, J. C. (1977). Oral communication apprehension: A summary of recent history and research. *Human Communication Research, 4,* 78–96.

McCrosky, J. C. (1978). Validity of the PRCA as an index of oral communication apprehension. *Communication Monographs, 45,* 192–203.

McCrosky, J. C. (1982). *An Introduction to Rhetorical Communication* (4th ed.). Englewood Cliffs, NJ: Prentice Hall.

Milhollan, F. & Forisha, B. E. (1972). *From Skinner to Rogers; Contrasting approaches to education.* Lincoln, NE: Professional Educators Publications, Inc.

Mineka, S. (1999, April). Psychological approaches to understanding anxiety disorders and their treatment. Keynote address at the Association for Applied Psychophysiology and Biofeedback meeting, Vancouver.

Nadon, R., Hoyt, I. P., Register, P. A., & Kihlstrom, J. F. (1991). Absorption and hypnotizability: Context effects reexamined. *Journal of Personality and Social Psychology, 60,* 144–153.

Ohman, A. (1986). Face the beast and fear the face: Animal and social fears as prototypes for evolutionary analyses of emotion. *Psychophysiology, 23,* 123–145.

Perez, F. (1997). *The biological basis of behavior.* Short course presented at the Association for Applied Psychophysiology and Feedback meeting, San Diego.

Perez, F. (2000). *Emotions and feelings in the bioregulation of consciousness.* Short course presented at the Association for Applied Psychophysiology and Feedback meeting, Denver.

Raleigh, M. J., McGuire, M. T., Brammer, G. A., Pollack, D. B., Yuwiller, A. (1991).Serotonergic mechanisms promote dominance acquisition in adult male vervet monkeys. *Brain Research, 559,* 181–190.

Restak, R. (1984). *Brain.* New York: Bantam.

Sagan, C. & Druyan, A. (1992). *Shadows of forgotten ancestors: A search for who we are.* New York: Random House.

Sapolsky, R. M. (1998). *Why zebras don't get ulcers.* New York: W. H. Freeman & Co.

Schore, A. (1994). *Affect regulation of the self: The neurobiology of emotional development.* Hillsdale, NJ: Laurence Erlbaum.

Schneier, F. & Welkowitz, L. (1996). *The hidden face of shyness.* New York: Avon Books.

Selye, H. (1956). *The stress of life.* New York: McGraw Hill.

Selye, H. (1974). *Stress without distress.* Philadelphia: Lippincott.

Thompson, J. G. (1988). *Psychobiology of emotions.* New York: Plenum Press.

Wickramasekera, I. (1988). *Clinical behavioral medicine: Some concepts and procedures.* New York: Plenum Press.

Wickramasekera, I. (1995). Somatization: Concepts, data, and predictions from the high risk model of threat perception. *Journal of Nervous and Mental Disease, 183,* 15–23.

Wickramasekera, I. (1998). Secrets kept from the mind but not the body or behavior: The unsolved problems of identifying and treating somatization and physiological disease. *Advances in Mind-Body Medicine, 14,* 81–132.

Zimbardo, P. G. (1977). *Shyness: What it is, what to do about it.* Reading, MA: Addison-Wesley.

Zimbardo, P. G., Pilkonis, P., & Norwood, R. (1975, May). The silent prison of shyness. *Psychology Today, 8,* 69–70, 72.

Suggested Reading

Barlow, D. (1988). *Anxiety and its disorders: The nature and treatment of anxiety and panic.* New York: Guilford Press.

Butcher, P., Elias A., & Raven R. (1993). *Psychogenic voice disorders and cognitive behaviour therapy.* London: Whurr Publishers.

Damasio, A. R. (1994). *Descarte's error: Emotion, reason, and the human brain.* New York: Avon Books.

Ekman, P. & Davidson, R. J. (Eds.). (1994). *The nature of emotion: Fundamental questions.* New York: Oxford University Press.

Everly, G. S., Jr. & Rosenfeld, R. (1981). *The nature and treatment of the stress response: A practical guide for clinicians.* New York: Plenum Press.

Goleman, D. (1995). *Emotional intelligence: Why it can matter more than IQ.* New York: Bantam Books.

Kagan, J. (1994). *Galen's prophecy: Temperament in human nature.* New York: Basic Books.

Kaplan, H. B. (Ed.). (1996). *Psychosocial stress: Perspectives on structure, theory, life-course, and methods.* San Diego: Academic Press.

Leary, M. R. & Kowalski, R. M. (1995). *Social anxiety.* New York: Guilford Press.

LeDoux, J. (1996). *The emotional brain: The mysterious underpinnings of emotional life.* New York: Simon & Schuster.

Marshall, J. R. (1994). *Social phobia: From shyness to stage fright.* New York: Basic Books.

Schneier, F. R. & Welkowitz, L. (1996). *The hidden face of shyness: Understanding and overcoming social anxiety.* New York: Avon Books.

Schore, A. (1994). *Affect regulation and the origin of the self: The neurobiology of emotional development.* Hillsdale, NJ: Laurence Erlbaum.

Selye, H. (1974). *Stress without distress.* Philadelphia: Lippincott.

Suter, S. (1986). *Health psychophysiology: Mind-body interactions in wellness and illness.* Hillsdale, NJ: Laurence Erlbaum Publishers.

Thompson, J. G. (1988). *The psychobiology of emotions.* New York: Plenum Press.

Wickramasekera, I. E. (1988). *Clinical behavioral medicine: Some concepts and procedures.* New York: Plenum Press.

Wickramasekera, I. E. (1998). Secrets kept from the mind but not the body or behavior: The unsolved problems of identifying and treating somatization and psychophysiological disease. *Advances in Mind-Body Medicine, 14,* 81–132.

CHAPTER

3

Psychological Perspectives

Anxiety Disorders

Identification and Intervention

Donald Moss, Ph.D.*

Anxiety is the total response of a human being to threat or danger. Each experience of anxiety involves a perception of danger, thoughts about harm, and a process of physiological alarm and activation. The accompanying behaviors display an emergency effort toward "fight or flight." The situation of threat may be mild, for example, when a golfer perceives that others will watch his or her golf swing, and the golfer fears that they may draw conclusions about the individual's athletic ability. Or the anxious situation may seem catastrophic, such as when an already lonely adolescent student recognizes that classmates can hear the youth stutter, and the youngster fears never having a friend. In each case, the experience of threat or danger is individualized—unique for each person at a given moment. The situation may look entirely safe and secure to others. For the anxious individual, however, each sensory modality goes "on alert" and focuses on the signs of possible harm.

*President of the Association for Applied Psychophysiology and Biofeedback, chief editor for *Biofeedback Newsmagazine*; consulting editor for *Journal of Neurotherapy*; partner in West Michigan Behavioral Health Services, Grand Haven and Muskegon, MI; adjunct graduate faculty member, of the Behavioral Medicine Research and Training Foundation, Suquamish, WA.

Fear and anxiety are universal human experiences that come and go in the course of life. Transient anxiety may accompany job loss, divorce, or a geographic move. In each case the fearful individual looks into the future and dreads an external catastrophe, but in a deeper sense the anxious person also experiences a threat to his or her own sense of identity (Fischer, 1970).

An anxiety disorder goes beyond normal, transient fears and anxiety (Coryell & Winokur, 1991; Emmelkamp, Bouman, & Scholing, 1992; Sheehan, 1983). An anxiety disorder involves a crippling and lingering process that disrupts the normal course of life. In the National Institute of Mental Health's Epidemiological Catchment Area survey, more than 25% of those surveyed identified themselves as "a nervous person." According to the same study, in any 6-month period, 8.9% of the population suffers an anxiety disorder, and about 14.6% of the population suffers an anxiety disorder in the course of their lifetimes. Anxiety disorders are twice as common in women (9.7% in a 1-month period) as in men (4.7% in a 1-month period). The population groups most vulnerable to anxiety disorders include: individuals 25 to 44 years old, female, separated and divorced, with low socioeconomic status (Regier, Narrow, & Rae, 1990). Nevertheless individuals of all ages, from early childhood to old age, are vulnerable to anxiety disorders.

Modern psychiatry and psychology have categorized the mental disorders in the American Psychiatric Association's *Diagnostic and Statistical Manual of Mental Disorders* (American Psychiatric Association, 1994). The fourth and most recent edition of this manual, known as DSM-IV, organizes all anxiety disorders into specific diagnostic categories with fairly clear, behavioral criteria for diagnosis. The most common of these disorders include panic disorder, the phobias, generalized anxiety disorder, and the "adjustment disorder with anxious features." Obsessive-compulsive disorder, posttraumatic stress disorder, and acute stress disorders also affect many individuals.

The Diagnosis of Anxiety
Why Is Diagnosis Important?

It is important to recognize the differences among the various anxiety disorders and to learn their diagnostic criteria, because current research shows that the conditions are different in behavioral pattern, natural history, and neurochemical basis. Some anxiety disorders, such as panic disorders, are transmitted largely by genetics, whereas others, such as posttraumatic stress disorder, are caused by a single traumatic event or series of traumatic events.

Because of such differences, each anxiety disorder must be recognized, treated, and managed differently. It is useful for speech-language pathologists to be familiar with the entire range of the anxiety disorders, but especially to understand the workings of social anxiety and social phobias, which can overlap so intimately with disorders of speech.

DSM-IV Anxiety Disorders

Brief summaries of the DSM-IV anxiety disorders follow.

Generalized Anxiety Disorder

Generalized anxiety disorder (GAD) is a persistent excessive fearfulness and worry that lingers at least 6 months and occurs more days than not. The individual reports fear and worry about a variety of situations, and not just one, as in many other anxiety disorders. For example, the individual may report a variety of fears about work, marriage, family, and health. The individual feels that he or she cannot control the worry. Restlessness, fatigue, irritability, muscle tension, and sleep disturbance accompany the worry. The fear and worry are disproportionate to the actual problems reported. The anxiety takes a toll over time, impairing ability to function at home, at work, and in social settings.

Generalized anxiety disorder is not diagnosed if the anxiety is caused by the direct physiological effects of a substance such as a drug, a medical condition such as hyperthyroidism, or another psychiatric disorder, such as a psychotic or paranoid ideas. The diagnosis of GAD includes the childhood equivalent disorder—overanxious disorder of childhood.

The Phobias

A phobia is any persistent, excessive, and irrational fear that goes beyond ordinary caution and concern. The phobias consist of both intense fearfulness and the accompanying avoidance patterns.

Specific Phobias

The specific phobias (formerly simple phobias) include fears of any specific object or situation, including animals (cats, dogs, mice, snakes), insects, lightning, heights, and flying. An individual with a specific phobia may suffer anticipatory anxiety, becoming fearful each time he or she expects to encounter the fearful object. Individuals will go to elaborate precautions to avoid contact with the feared object or situation. A 40-year-old Michigan man with a fear of flying drove alone

26 hours in each direction from Michigan to Colorado several weekends each winter to meet his friends at ski resorts rather than face his flying phobia.

Agoraphobia

The more complex phobias include agoraphobia, which is a generalized fear of places or situations from which escape may be difficult or embarrassing. Anticipating exposure to such situations triggers either a panic attack or panic-like anxiety. The anxiety often spreads to a number of related situations and may become pervasive, with only a slight sense of refuge in the individual's home or in a room of the home. An individual may make a great effort to avoid the anxiety-provoking situations or will endure the situations with distress and anxiety.

Because agoraphobia so often involves panic attacks and occurs often in the context of panic disorder, the following three diagnostic variations clarify the relationship between the two disorders in a particular individual: agoraphobia without history of panic disorder, panic disorder with agoraphobia, or panic disorder without agoraphobia.

Social Phobia

A social phobia is a persistent and pronounced fear of social situations and performance situations in which embarrassment may occur. An individual typically seeks to avoid or minimize contact with social and performance situations. Each time the individual encounters such a situation, anxiety almost invariably occurs. Sometimes the anxiety is a full-blown panic attack and sometimes it is an intense nervousness without panic. The social anxiety is accompanied by physical symptoms such as sweating, trembling, blushing, heart palpitations, and tremors. These physical symptoms often then become the focus of further anxiety. Performance anxiety is a major symptom of social phobia and has been discussed in Chapters 1 and 2.

For a diagnosis of social phobia, the symptoms must disrupt an individual's life, his or her job, school functioning, normal routine, or social activities. Social phobia is discussed at greater length later in this chapter.

Panic Disorder

A panic attack is an overwhelming experience of terror and dread. Panic is typically accompanied by rapid respiration, shortness of breath, rapid and irregular heart rate, profuse sweating, chest pain or discomfort, nausea, a sense of trembling and jitteriness, and racing thoughts. Individuals often report some specific and overwhelming fear—of dying, going crazy, or losing control of one's actions.

Panic disorder is diagnosed when panic attacks become more frequent, at least four occurring in 4 months, and when one or more panic attacks occur out of the blue, without any detectable trigger. An individual must also suffer at least four of the typical symptoms of panic within 10 minutes of the onset of the panic. Panic disorder co-occurs so often with agoraphobia (described previously), that panic disorder is now coded diagnostically as "with agoraphobia" or "without agoraphobia."

Obsessive-Compulsive Disorder

Obsessive-compulsive disorder (OCD) is a condition marked by recurrent obsessions and compulsions that are severe enough to disrupt normal life. Obsessions are ideas, impulses, or images that persist against an individual's wishes and cause anxiety and distress. The ideas are experienced as irrational, inappropriate, and intrusive. Typical obsessions include preoccupation with germs and dirt; concern with bodily symptoms, waste, and secretions; fears of harm to oneself or others; fears of something terrible happening; fears of committing embarrassing acts; and extreme religious preoccupation.

Compulsions are repetitive behaviors that aim to reduce a person's anxiety. The individual feels driven to continue the behavior to reduce distress or escape threatening events. Typical compulsions include cleaning and washing rituals, repetitive checking behaviors, the compulsion to repeat certain actions or gestures, an urge to order and arrange things, repetitive touching and counting, excessive hoarding and collecting, and excessive seeking of medical reassurance for bodily complaints (Greist & Jefferson, 1995).

Posttraumatic Stress Disorder

Posttraumatic stress disorder (PTSD) is an often-disabling condition resulting from exposure to extremely traumatic events of a real or perceived threat to one's own life or well-being or to those of others. Typical events triggering PTSD include combat in wartime, rape and assault, auto accident, house fires, and cumulative exposure to brutal accidents and injuries. The result of the traumatic experience is a recurrent experience of fear, helplessness, and horror. The individual with PTSD reexperiences the painful event(s) vividly, in flashbacks, dreams, nightmares, and reenactments, as though the event(s) was/were actually happening. The individual shows a persisting physiological arousal and vigilance, accompanied by sleep disturbance, irritability, poor concentration, and/or exaggerated startle response.

A variety of cognitive (mental) changes also occur with PTSD. The individual perceives the surrounding world as menacing and not welcoming, and perceives his or her personal future as "foreshortened." Any reminders of the trauma-event can trigger a physiological and emotional emergency state. The individual with PTSD often engages in pervasive efforts to avoid any person, activity, or situation related to the original trauma, and may show a general numbing of emotional life, detachment from loved ones, and loss of interest in once favored activities. PTSD is diagnosed only if the symptoms persist for 3 months or more and significantly disrupt an individual's vocational, social, and personal functioning. The disorder is labeled as "delayed" if the onset of symptoms occurs at least 6 months after the precipitating event.

Acute Stress Disorder

Acute stress disorder (ASD) is an immediate and shorter-term version of posttraumatic stress disorder. ASD is diagnosed if the symptoms develop within 4 weeks of the traumatic event, and only if the symptoms last for a minimum of 2 days and remit within 4 weeks. Otherwise the triggers, symptoms, and long-lasting transformations of an individual's physiology and emotional life are the same as PTSD.

Adjustment Disorder with Anxiety

An adjustment disorder is a disturbance in mood or behavior with onset within 3 months of some stressful life event, and ceasing within 6 months after the stressful life event ends. When the predominant symptom is anxiety, the symptoms may include nervousness, worry, and jitteriness. The anxiety must disrupt daily life, and fail to meet the criteria for other DSM-IV disorders. The disturbance may be classified as acute (lasting less than 6 months) or chronic (when the stressor itself persists, and the symptoms therefore persist for more than 6 months).

Screening for Anxiety Disorders

The majority of patients with anxiety disorders present in primary care medicine, often with physical complaints, but often the anxiety disorder is not diagnosed. When anxiety disorders are present and untreated, interventions for the comorbid medical disorder are less successful. Other individuals with anxiety disorders request behavioral services, but often for relationship conflict, job stress, or other psychosocial complaints. Others with anxiety disorders seek speech and language therapy. Many in each group will fail to receive effective treatment because the background anxiety problem is not identified.

Health care and speech-language clinicians can improve detection by asking key questions and monitoring for central signs and symptoms. The questions in Table 3-1 will not provide conclusive diagnostic information, but answers should alert the health professional to the probable presence of an anxiety disorder. With such probability, a more complete examination is warranted.

TABLE 3-1. Screening Questions for the Anxiety Disorders

Screening for Panic Disorder	Screening for Agoraphobia	Screening for OCD
Do you have attacks of overwhelming fear and terror? Sometimes out of the blue without a trigger?	Are you anxious about being in certain places and situations, from which escape may be difficult?	Do you have troubling thoughts that won't stop, no matter how hard you try?
Do you have fears of dying, heart attack, going crazy, or losing control?	Do you avoid many places which you associate with anxiety and fear?	Do you keep things extremely clean and orderly, or wash your hands more frequently than other people?
Do you have racing, pounding heart, sweating, trembling, and rapid breathing during attacks (in the absence of organic illness)?		Do you check things repeatedly and to excess?
Do you worry about having another attack?		Does it often take you much longer than others to complete simple tasks?

(continues)

TABLE 3-1. *continued*

Screening for PTSD	Screening for Specific Phobia	Screening for Social Phobia
Were you physically or sexually abused, assaulted, or involved in a shocking event that continues to bother you?	Do you have fears of contact with specific objects or situations?	Do you have persisting fears of social or performance situations?
Do you have painful memories, nightmares, or flashbacks to traumatic event(s)?	Do you go to elaborate lengths to avoid such objects or situations?	Do you avoid or dread social situations?
Do you sometimes relive the shocking event as though it were happening now?		Do social fears disrupt your life?
Do things happen in the present which take you back to a painful past event(s)?		

Screening for Generalized Anxiety Disorder	Screening for Adjustment Disorder with Anxiety
Do you have troubling fears and worries more days than not, in many or all situations?	Are you experiencing anxiety (nervousness, worry, or jitteriness) in response to stressful life events?
Is it difficult for you to control your worries?	Did the anxiety commence within three months of the events, and persist no more than six months after the event ends?
Are you frequently tense, restless, strained or irritable?	Is the anxiety disrupting your daily life?
Have your fears and worries persisted for six months, and do they disrupt your ability to function in everyday life?	

Comorbidity of Anxiety Disorders and Depression

In spite of the emphasis on identifying the diverse anxiety disorders, diagnostic distinctions are never absolute. Many individuals show symptoms of more than one anxiety disorder or report depressive symptoms that accompany their anxiety. For example 33% of persons with social phobia also report symptoms of generalized anxiety disorder, 8% report simple phobias and 2% report panic disorder (Turner, Beidel, Borden, Stanley, & Jacob, 1991). In addition, 6% of persons with social phobias also report symptoms of dysthymic disorder (neurotic depression) or major depressive disorder (Turner et al., 1991). Research has also shown that the DSM-IV diagnostic categories are not discrete. There is a significant overlap between the symptoms of social phobia and those of avoidant personality disorder (Holt, Heimberg, & Hope, 1992; Turner, Beidel, & Townsley, 1992; Widiger, 1992).

The Natural History of the Anxiety Disorders

The natural history of an illness or morbid condition includes the typical age of onset, the manner of onset, the typical course, and the likelihood of any resolution during the individual's life cycle. Anxiety disorders vary greatly in their typical age of onset. Notice the frequent early ages of onset for obsessive-compulsive disorder (early childhood) and social phobia (late childhood). The commonsense belief that most children "have nothing to worry about" is misguided, as individuals with anxiety disorders may worry and experience fearfulness whether or not there are objective problems in the family and environment. (See Table 3-2.)

TABLE 3-2. Onset of the DSM-IV Anxiety Disorders

Anxiety Disorder	Typical Age of Onset
Generalized anxiety disorder	Usually 20s or 30s
Panic disorder with or without agoraphobia	Late 20s
Agoraphobia without panic disorder	20s or 30s
Social phobia	Late childhood, early teens
Simple phobia	Late 40s (except for highly specific fears such as driving)
Obsessive compulsive disorder	Childhood, to young adult
Posttraumatic stress disorder	Onset at any age, following trauma

Progression of an Anxiety Disorder

Onset of Anxiety

The initial onset of anxiety disorders varies greatly. Some patients can date their anxiety to a specific date and situation. This is always the case with posttraumatic stress disorder, in which, by definition, the trigger is a remarkable traumatic incident. In many cases, patients with panic disorder and phobias can point to a specific situation or series of situations that triggered their first episodes. Later episodes of panic or phobic symptoms, however, may occur out of the blue, without any apparent trigger or be triggered by new situations. The original cause of the first episode becomes less closely associated with succeeding episodes.

In contrast, many patients with generalized anxiety disorder or obsessive-compulsive disorder describe a gradual occurrence and increase in anxiety. Stressful events may bring on new episodes, or worsen symptoms, but no single stressor can explain the course of the disorder.

Anticipatory Anxiety

In anticipatory anxiety, once an individual has experienced anxiety episodes, he or she begins to experience an increasingly constant fear of the next episode and to fear of any situation that might trigger the next episode. This is anticipatory anxiety—a vigilant fear of another attack. This anticipatory fear can arouse the physiology of anxiety and trigger the next episode. Because of this anticipatory anxiety, a wide variety of events can serve to trigger the next episode of anxiety for the vulnerable individual. Physical exertion, a startling event, illness and fatigue, a racing heartbeat or rapid breathing, or a situation in which one has been anxious before can all trigger anxiety.

Cognitive Escalation of Anxiety

Once the individual with cognitive escalation of anxiety begins to perceive a threat and to react with fearfulness, a serious anxiety episode becomes a possibility. However, a number of intervening steps must take place, to escalate the initial lower-level fearfulness into a full-scale anxiety attack. Some of the escalation takes place because the individual senses his or her initial anxiety and begins to have anxious thoughts: "Oh, no. It's happening again," or "I'm having another attack, I know it," or "I'll never stop having these attacks." Such thoughts, in turn, trigger more physical arousal, including such symptoms as rapid or irregular heartbeat, rapid uneven breathing, fluttery feelings in the chest, or dizzy or nauseous sensations. The rapid breathing is especially important because hyperventilation changes the balance of carbon dioxide and oxygen in the body, triggering cardiovascular irregularities, inducing dizziness, and lightheadedness, and producing many additional sensations of unreality and physical unease (Timmons & Ley, 1994).

Symptomatic Focus

Once an individual notices increasing physical sensations of anxiety, additional fearful thoughts can take over and produce a more heightened anxiety: "Oh my God, I'm having a heart attack," or "I'm losing my mind," or "I'm out of control, and there's nothing I can do." The more the individual focuses on symptoms, the more severe become the subjective fears and the physiological activation. Focusing on the symptoms does not bring resolution, but rather escalation.

Increasing Chronicity

Many of the anxiety disorders are "remitting and relapsing conditions." This means that individuals will experience episodes of worsened symptoms followed by times in which the individual is symptom-free or nearly so. However, one also frequently sees a progression from intermittent anxiety to constant, incessant anxiety without relief. Intermittent physiological activation becomes chronic activation. Intermittent anticipatory anxiety becomes constant fear of the next episode. Eventually there may be no respite, and the individual feels trapped inside one long never-ending attack.

Psychophysiology and the Escalation of Anxiety

Individuals with GAD (chronically fearful "worry-warts") or PTSD (survivors of catastrophically traumatic events) typically show a state of chronic hyperarousal. Such individuals show an elevated basal heart rate and respiration rate, chronically tense musculature, and/or a state of emotional tension and sensory vigilance. In other words, their bodies are overactivated all of the time, not just when they have a flashback or intrusive memory. In such persons who are consistently anxious over time, the changes in the brain, nervous system, and endocrine system become dramatic. For example, research on Vietnam veterans, rape victims, and other survivors of traumatic events, shows that the *locus coeruleus* in the brainstem becomes chronically overactivated after such emotionally traumatic events and blocks any efforts of the individual to calm himself or herself emotionally and feel normal again (van der Kolk, 1987). Even when the person's surroundings are placid, such individuals live as though about to reenter a life-threatening battle.

Similarly, many patients with panic disorder show a greater sensitization to anxiety over time; at any moment, the slightest trigger brings on a rapid flaring of subjective terror and a physiologic alarm response. Their physiological activation loses its episodic character, and becomes one of constant arousal with higher peaks during an "episode."

Researchers have described this "kindling effect" as common following repeated exposure to intense anxiety (van der Kolk & Greenberg, 1987). It takes progressively less real threat or danger to "kindle" a new fearful or panic experience in such hyperaroused individuals. Thus the Vietnam vet initially may have reacted only to a new exposure to combat, but over time comes to respond with dramatic flashbacks and terror to any loud sound or sudden movement or even to smells reminiscent of the war zone.

Physiologically, anxiety describes a wide range of human experiences, ranging from normal uneasiness at facing a new situation to the raw terror relived by the rape victim each time she senses that someone may be following her. The person experiencing recurrent or chronic anxieties will show increasing physiological changes: chronic hyperarousal and vigilance and/or a susceptibility to rapid kindling of extreme states of fear and terror. The common-sense advice to "calm down" or "get a grip" has little impact on individuals living through such extremes of emotional and physiological arousal.

Avoidance Behavior

As anxiety episodes proliferate, the individual often avoids the original scene of anxiety episodes, for fear of triggering new anxiety. Over time such avoidance generalizes beyond the original scene of anxiety to include avoidance of any situation resembling such scenes, or any situation reminding one in the faintest way of past episodes. The individual initially may avoid one supermarket where a panic attack occurred, but eventually will avoid all supermarkets, all stores, and all public places. The anxiety sufferer's personal world becomes progressively more restricted over time, and at the extreme many individuals never leave the subjective safety and comfort of their home.

With progressive restriction of activity, many individuals also lose confidence. The avoidance behavior removes any opportunity to master their fears and regain confidence. Over time, the individual experiences a generalized feeling of powerlessness.

Anxiety Is a Threshold Phenomenon

Even when genetic involvement is clear and when neurobiological mechanisms can be identified, as in obsessive-compulsive disorder and panic disorder, the anxiety episodes can be triggered by a time of acute life stress. We can speak of a "threshold" for anxiety, such that the accumulation of stress exceeds the threshold of the individual's coping skills. This moment triggers the intense attack of anxiety and terror. Over time, the threshold wears lower, as an individual's coping resources erode, and it takes less and less of a trigger to bring on an attack of acute anxiety. Temporary conditions can also erode coping and lower the threshold for anxiety episodes. Illness and sleep deprivation both render individuals more vulnerable to anxiety episodes.

On the other hand, the relation between life-stress and anxiety episodes isn't always clear. Many individuals perceive life as more overwhelming once anxiety commences. During the anxiety episode, an individual fails to cope with stressful situations that the person would have handled well at other times. A vicious cycle develops, and the individual attributes his or her episode to stress, when the emergence of anxiety was already underway when the life stress occurred.

Comprehensive Treatment of Anxiety

In this section, the general framework for effective treatment of anxiety disorders is examined, and specific interventions for social anxiety and social phobias reviewed. The frame of reference is a comprehensive bioinformational theory of anxiety that integrates cognitive, behavioral, and physiological aspects of the anxiety experience for unified structural understanding (Foa & Kozak, 1998). Many of the treatment interventions useful for individuals with anxiety disorder involve mastering specific skills. Learning about these useful skills enables a speech-language pathologist to play a helpful role with the mildly to moderately anxious patient, and to recognize when the more severely anxious patient should be referred for specialized treatment.

Framework for Intervention: The Three Components of Anxiety

Peter Lang has emphasized that there are three distinct components of anxiety: (1) subjective fear, (2) physiological activation, and (3) avoidance behavior (cited by Rachman, 1982, 1999). These three components do not covary on a reliable basis. The three components are loosely coupled and, at times, discordant. An individual may express extreme subjective fear, yet show little autonomic/physiologic reactivity. The three components of anxiety are also not synchronous. That is, they do

not always change at the same rate. It is common, for example, for phobic patients to report success in resuming driving or returning to public
places, yet still report that "by the way, doctor, I'm still really afraid."

This distinction is useful for treatment, because treatment may be
targeted at any one of several distinct components. Effective physiological interventions train an individual to reduce physiological activation
through biofeedback and various relaxation skills. Each method of
relaxation leads to a self-quieting of the body and a reduction in the
physiology of stress and alarm. But the individual may still report fearful thoughts and feelings and hesitate to enter anxiety-provoking situations (Rachman, 1982, 1999).

Effective behavioral therapy prepares a patient to not run away
behaviorally from anxiety-provoking situations. This training enables a
patient to manage, but not eliminate, subjective fear. In many cases, a
patient becomes confident about entering and handling a situation, but
still shows measurable physiological arousal and reports subjective
fear. The perception of danger persists and the physiological alarm
response continues, while the individual gains behavioral confidence.

Finally, cognitive therapy teaches patients to modify fearful
thoughts, redirect attention away from fears, and self-coach themselves
to overcome fearful experiences. Yet physiological activation and
behavioral avoidance may persist.

Ultimately, complete recovery requires change in three areas: the
cognitive-affective experience of fear, physiological activation, and
behavioral avoidance. However, treatment for any given anxious individual may emphasize one or another dimension more than the others,
and the sequence of optimal interventions may also vary from one
course of treatment to the next (Knapp & VandeCreek, 1994).

Patient Education: The Active Mastery Orientation

One of the keys to success in treating individuals with serious anxiety
disorders is patient education. It is necessary for a patient to reframe
his or her understanding of anxiety to enable the patient to believe in
the efficacy of a new approach to recovery. The cognitive-behavioral
and psychophysiological approaches to anxiety disorders are founded
on an active mastery model.

In the active mastery model, an individual acquires knowledge about
anxiety and self-regulation skills. The knowledge and skills support developing active coping mechanisms for each anxiety episode. The acquisition
of knowledge and skills by the client and growing self-confidence in his or
her actions combine to reduce anticipation and terror about a potential

future attack, which, in turn, erodes the triggering mechanisms for anxiety. This active coping accumulates and supports a new confidence. The confidence initially is based on belief in an approach, but eventually becomes "self-efficacy"—a belief in oneself. Initially, an individual may only believe that he or she is merely capable of withstanding and surviving an anxiety episode, but eventually the individual becomes confident of triumphing over anxiety.

Albert Bandura (1997) described two stages in the development of self-efficacy. First, the individual must learn and come to believe that other persons can overcome a problem or accomplish a task. Second, the individual must learn and come to believe that he himself or she herself can overcome a problem or accomplish a task.

In applying this self-efficacy framework to anxiety disorders, the first step is for the patient to understand that many other individuals facing equally overwhelming anxiety have learned skills that enabled them to overcome their anxiety disorder. Bibliotherapy is helpful, because the patient can read about how others learned skills and overcame their anxiety disorder. Psychoeducational group-based treatment can also be helpful, because all patients can observe others mastering skills and gaining confidence.

The second step is for a patient to come to believe that he himself or she herself can master skills and overcome an anxiety disorder. The optimal strategy is to present the patient with small, achievable steps, providing the opportunity for small successes. Biofeedback, for example, provides the opportunity for an individual to reduce muscle tension or deepen breathing, gaining a sense of control over his or her own physiology in a safe setting. This mastery can be gradually extended to build confidence in physiological and subjective control in threatening situations that once triggered panic.

Cognitive self-help procedures can be used in combination with biofeedback to further create voluntary control skills and to extend self-efficacy. Many patients report a true "eureka!"[1] experience when they begin to recognize the mind-body connection. For example, a patient who deliberately begins to visualize a frightening situation or to deliberately engage in fearful thoughts, may be shocked to see the biofeedback instrument register an increase in muscle tension, an increase in heart rate, and an increase in the rate and irregularity of respiration: "You mean, what I think in my mind affects my body?"

---

[1] Exclamation attributed to Archimedes on discovering a way to determine the purity of gold.

A final step in patient education is to shift the patient's focus from any fearful situation "out there," to the personal experience of fear, accompanied by activated physiology and fearful thoughts. It is the experience of fear that is the true nemesis, and the external events often so intimately associated with anxiety are merely the triggers. Once a patient comes to recognize that he or she is primarily afraid of anxious feelings and thinking, the process of self-mastery and anxiety management can begin.

Physiological Quieting
The Stress Response and the Relaxation Response

When a human being perceives danger, the human organism displays a series of changes called the stress response, including: tense muscles, elevated heart rate and blood pressure, rapid respiration, anxious vigilant thinking, a suppressed immune system, and increased output of adrenaline and blood sugar. These stress-related changes fatigue the body and undermine health (Everly, 1989).

Experiences of relaxation create effects opposite to stress, which is called the relaxation response. The relaxation response reverses the negative effects of stress on the human body. Respiration becomes slower and deeper, heart rate and blood pressure decrease, muscles relax, the immune system works more effectively, and thinking becomes more open and relaxed (Benson, 1975).

Long-term cultivation of the relaxation response reduces an individual's anxiety and distress and enhances subjective well-being. Long-term practice of relaxation creates a quiet, open mental state, with spontaneous creativity and moderates extreme emotional states.

How Can the Relaxation Response Be Created?

Many normal human activities can bring on the relaxation response: a relaxed walk along the beach, listening to soothing music, practicing a craft, or working quietly in a garden. However, many times human beings believe they are relaxed, while some physiological system in their body remains tense or over-activated. It is important to learn self-quieting skills that relax one's entire body and mind.

Self-Quieting Skills

The most reliable way to induce the relaxation response is to learn relaxation or meditation skills. There are hundreds of different methods for creating physical and emotional relaxation. Each method teaches a kind of voluntary control.

- **Autogenic relaxation:** Autogenic training involves listening to a series of phrases describing the sensations of heaviness, looseness, warmth and inner peace accompanying relaxation. As the phrases work on the body, the individual enters a deep state of mental and physical relaxation.
- **Calm scene:** One of the simplest forms of relaxation is to picture oneself in a peaceful, comfortable place, and use the power of the imagination to experience the soothing effects of being in that imagined place on the body and mind.
- **Diaphragmatic breathing:** Breathing fully and slowly, from the diaphragm, brings about deep relaxation and many powerful physiological changes in the body and nervous system. Paced, deep breathing is a part of many religious schools of meditation, because it creates inner serenity.
- **Slow correct diaphragmatic breathing:** Five to seven breaths per minute (BPM) is the most effective way to enhance respiratory sinus arrhythmia (RSA), the measure of synchrony between the respiratory and cardiovascular systems. Slower diaphragmatic breathing and enhanced RSA result in a decreased heart rate and greater homeostasis in the autonomic nervous system, thereby reducing anxiety symptoms.
- **Meditation:** There are many meditation techniques. Each type of meditation focuses the mind and creates serenity within. Regular meditation also relaxes the body and has powerful health benefits.
- **Progressive muscle relaxation:** The individual alternately tenses and relaxes each muscle group throughout the body. Tensing the muscles first increases an individual's ability to release the tension. Observing the contrast between tense and relaxed muscles increases personal awareness of tension when it develops in everyday life.
- **Passive muscle relaxation:** This brief relaxation method quickly relaxes muscle groups throughout the body. This method avoids the tensing step of progressive muscle relaxation and is easier for patients with chronic pain to tolerate.
- **Visualization:** Visualization involves picturing a series of images that induce peacefulness, physical healing, pain relief, and other health enhancing effects.

Daily Practice of Relaxation Skills

The regular practice of relaxation exercises for 20 to 30 minutes daily can produce a generalized calming effect throughout one's life. General guidelines for relaxation follow.

Instruction: Choose a time of day that will consistently best allow you to practice new skills. Select a quiet environment with a comfortable chair. Mentally let go of any problems and distractions. For the moment in time of a relaxation exercise, you need not solve any life-problems. You need only enjoy the process of physical, emotional, and spiritual relaxation.

As you master new skills, begin performing brief "minirelaxation" exercises in the course of the day. Relax for 2 or 5 minutes, and then go on with your activity. This will generalize the benefits of your relaxation to a variety of settings in your life. Most persons who do daily relaxation exercises feel calmer wherever they are and whatever they are doing. Many persons who relax regularly find that they cope better with problems, let go of problems more quickly, and react less extremely when troubles arise. When you experience tension under stress, imagine your last experience of relaxation, and you will rapidly recover a relaxed state.

Biofeedback

Biofeedback is a method for learning better awareness and control over one's own mind and body. Biofeedback instruments are electronic instruments designed to monitor change in the human body and to provide simultaneous feedback to the user. By watching a feedback display, the user becomes more aware of physical and mental changes taking place and gains control over changing his or her own mind and body. Almost any bodily process that can be monitored electronically can be used for biofeedback training. Today, common devices measure muscle activity, hand temperature, nervous activation, blood pressure, heart rate, brain wave activity, respiration, and brain blood flow.

Biofeedback is especially helpful in relaxation training. Many persons will inform the therapist that they feel relaxed, but the biofeedback instrument will show that there is a continuation of excessive muscle tension and nervous activity, elevated blood pressure, and overvigilant brain activity. By monitoring a person during relaxation, a therapist can guide the individual to relax all physiological systems.

Several biofeedback modalities can help in relaxation training. For example, thermal biofeedback is often achieved through the use of a handheld thermometer to help an individual learn to self-warm his or her hands, which leads to relaxation and a dilation of the arteries carrying warm blood to the hands. With respiratory biofeedback the individual can learn to breathe fully, smoothly, and slowly, creating deep mental and physical relaxation of the body. Paced diaphragmatic breathing also reverses the physiological effects of hyperventilation, which play a central role in many patients with panic disorder. EMG (electromyography) can help people identify and reduce muscular tensions. EEG (electroencephalography) biofeedback (or neurofeedback) is used to teach an individual to enter an "alpha brain state," in which the person is physically and mentally more relaxed, calm, mentally alert, and yet open to whatever is happening. A portable GSR (galvanic skin response) instrument can feed back information on sweat gland activity and pore size, a direct measure of the sympathetic nervous system, which is chemically activated during stress. The Cardiosignalizer,™ a Russian device that simultaneously measures diaphragmatic breathing and heart rate can also be used for anxiety reduction.

Once an individual achieves a relaxed state, muscle tension, nervous activity, heart rate, breathing rate and/or blood pressure decrease, while finger temperature increases and the brain produces more activity in the "alpha" range. Each of these changes is beneficial in restoring balance to the human body, allowing body organs to function in better harmony.

Applying Relaxation and Biofeedback Skills to Anxiety and Anxiety Attacks

Initially it is helpful for an anxious individual to employ relaxation skills "just for practice" in quiet, nonanxious times. Once a relaxed state is achieved, the individual can deliberately trigger anxiety by visualizing a threatening situation, imagining his or her own physiological symptoms of anxiety, and calling to mind the most fearful thoughts from anxiety attacks. The individual can watch his or her physiological response to anxiety on the biofeedback display and then resume relaxation exercises to restore the relaxed state. Repeatedly inducing anxiety and restoring relaxation during relaxation practice or during biofeedback sessions increases an individual's ability to master real-life attacks of anxiety.

Later, when the skills have been strengthened, it is time to begin relaxing during anxious moments. Initially one sets the goal of relaxing in spite of anxiety. This instructional set dispels unrealistic hopes that the relaxation exercise will immediately banish all traces of anxiety. However, if an individual gradually develops the ability to relax in spite of anxiety and, thus, succeeds in moderating several of the physiological concomitants of anxiety, then he or she is accumulating mastery over anxiety. These skills also increase an individual's readiness to deliberately seek out anxious situations.

Anxiety Challenge Trials in the Office and in situ Experiences

Many patients can trigger an anxiety episode in the office by imagining a feared situation, touching or handling a dreaded object, hyperventilating, spinning on a rotating stool, or walking rapidly on a step machine. The choice of the method to induce anxiety depends on the typical triggers for anxiety and the typical components in the patient's anxiety episode. If exertion and elevated heart rate are typical triggers, then, of course, exertion in the office will usually induce anxiety. If vertigo and dizziness are typical components of an anxiety episode, then spinning on a stool or chair will frequently induce anxiety. If hyperventilation is a typical component in an anxiety episode, then guiding the patient to take in large-volume deep breaths for 1 minute will typically induce recognizable symptoms of an anxiety episode (Conway, 1994). If an individual compulsively uses a glove to touch doorknobs, then touching the doorknob can be a useful tool to induce the anxiety.

When a patient can induce the anxiety in a controlled office situation on a repeated basis and practice self-quieting, the sense of self-mastery is greatly enhanced. For the first time a patient ceases to be a victim and truly experiences him- or herself as actively engaging the anxiety. It is helpful to prepare the patient with thorough mastery of solid self-quieting and self-talk skills before attempting the anxiety-challenge trials. Nevertheless, many individuals will benefit from the repeated exposure, even without using any specific coping skills. Once a patient has mastered anxiety in the office setting, then he or she is ready to progressively seek out more and more difficult anxiogenic situations in everyday life. The next section on behavioral modification explores the use of an anxiety hierarchy.

Behavioral Modification

The primary objective of behavioral modification in the anxiety disorders is to restore the full range of normal behaviors and to confront avoidance behaviors. A helpful tool is the construction of a hierarchy of anxiety-provoking situations, including any and all situations that an individual avoids. A hierarchy is like a ladder or staircase. Human beings cannot tackle their most frightening situations all at once.

Approaching one's most anxious situation one small step at a time makes progress possible.

To construct a hierarchy the patient is instructed to list on paper situations (places, activities, or social settings) that trigger even the slightest anxiety or fearfulness. Figure 5-4 is an example of a form that can be used by clients to make lists. Once the individual has mostly completed the list, the situations should be ranked from the bottom (least anxiety provoking) to the top (most anxiety provoking). The situations at the bottom of the hierarchy may be settings the individual knows he or she can handle, although with mild discomfort. The situations at the top of the hierarchy may include settings that the patient cannot ever imagine trying to deal with.

The hierarchy then guides an individual into the single most effective form of behavior therapy, what is called exposure therapy, or systematic desensitization. An individual bravely brings him- or herself to move up the ladder. The individual first tackles situations at the bottom of the list and then proceeds up the hierarchy to more difficult tasks, using self-talk and relaxation skills to manage anxiety as he or she proceeds to face new situations. The purpose is twofold: first, for the individual to recover access to a full range of places and activities in everyday life and, second, to reinforce the personal experience of mastery over anxiety. As an individual proceeds upward through the hierarchy, each situation becomes desensitized. The situation can no longer readily trigger an alarming anxiety. That which was once traumatic can become everyday and banal.

Cognitive Change

The previous section on the escalation of anxiety highlighted the role of fearful thoughts in escalating the intensity of anxiety. Regardless of the initial trigger for an individual's fears and anxieties, fearful thoughts play a major role in the escalation and maintenance of anxiety. Barlow (1994); Beck and Emery (1985); and Foa, Franklin, Perry, and Herbert (1996) have identified distorted and maladaptive patterns of thinking that contribute to the severity and chronicity of anxiety. In the following, several common cognitive strategies for managing and mastering anxiety are reviewed.

Reassurance

One of the first cognitive interventions for most persons is reassurance. Initially, the anxious individual with physical complaints will benefit from realistic medical reassurance. The primary care physician is usually in the best position to conduct a thorough physical examination, including blood work and then to reassure the individual that there are no indications of heart disease or other medical illness causing the person's symptoms. This reassurance is only successful if the physician conducts a thorough exam to ensure that there are not conditions such as abnormal thyroid function, hypoglycemia, menopause or other hormonal fluctuation, or caffeine or nicotine abuse that could account for the anxiety symptoms (Gold, 1989). In cases of voice or speech disorders, laryngologists or other appropriate specialists should provide physical examinations to ensure that there are no medical conditions that interfere with normal function and to provide reassurance to the patient.

Following a medical workup, an individual can be reassured that his or her physical and mental symptoms, which should be specifically listed and explained, are normal accompaniments of anxiety. Then the patient will better accept that these symptoms present no risk for health, and that they will fade with mastery over the anxiety.

Once the patient has accepted medical reassurance, the stage is set for self-reassurance. Many individuals encounter recurrent fears of illness long after their physicians have identified anxiety as the primary diagnosis. In such cases the individual needs to coach him- or herself, using self-talk to assuage fears:

- "My racing heart and flushed feelings are normal symptoms of anxiety."
- "If I can sit back and deepen my breathing, I'll feel so much better."
- "My life is not in danger, as my recent exam showed."
- "These symptoms will pass shortly, and I'll then go on with my day."
- "I'm not going to faint; it's my breathing that makes me feel that way."

Floating

Claire Weeks (1978) developed and popularized a strategy that she calls floating. When the first symptoms of anxiety surface, the patient needs to consider floating through the rest of the episode. Floating means that one accepts the anxiety, reminds oneself that it will be of no harm, and steps back to observe the process as it happens. Dr. Weeks suggests that floating is the opposite of fighting. When floating, an individual won't become agitated and fearful that "Oh my God, I'm getting anxious again." Instead, the person floats through the anxiety and past it or allows it to float and flow past him or her. This acceptance dilutes the potential intensity of anxiety symptoms.

To master floating, the client is told to remind oneself that anxiety is a benign process—that anxiety is very uncomfortable, but won't harm one. In addition, the patient is reminded that when one lets go and accepts the onset of anxiety, one dulls its sting. The letting go attitude reduces inner turmoil about what might happen in the future. Over time, floating allows small anxieties to remain small, without escalating into a panic attack.

Patient as Scientist Model

When anxiety attacks, an individual becomes subjectively absorbed with symptoms and fears. The anxious individual loses the big picture and finds it difficult to keep symptoms and situations in any kind of objective perspective. The overwhelming fearfulness of acute anxiety can undermine even the best reassurance by physicians and counselors.

The cognitive psychologist George Kelly (personal communication, Adams-Webber & Macuso, 1983; Kelly, 1955, 1963; Pervin, 1975; von Scheele, December, 18, 1999) developed a model that invites the individual to act and think in the manner of a scientist. Kelly and his students recognized that human beings become trapped not by objective forces, but by their own cognitive constructions about reality. However, human beings can also free themselves by observing, studying, and reconstructing their reality. Applying this "man as a scientist" perspective to the anxiety disorders, it is not the external event—the elevator, the crowded store, or the social setting—that threatens to overwhelm the person, but his or her fears about the event, attributions to the event, and mental constructions about the event.

A cognitive therapist can teach an anxious patient to make accurate behavioral observations, keep symptom logs, and fill out daily worksheets for skills the person has practiced. Objective self-observation is a helpful mental model for approaching each moment of anxiety. The individual can substitute a new objective focus for the previous subjective absorption, posing such questions as:

- What aspects of this situation seem to be triggering my fears?
- What negative interpretations and fears are escalating my anxiety?
- How well am I relaxing my physiology now? Can I breathe more fully and regularly? Can I relax my muscles more completely?
- If I focus on getting through this situation, can I remain longer than last time?

Each time an anxious individual ventures into a potentially anxiogenic situation can be viewed as a scientific experiment, with potential for learning. This reframing of one's activities as objective experiments gives new significance to both behavioral successes and behavioral failures. Each new effort at coping with anxiety represents an experiment from which one can draw new conclusions about which specific skill most successfully moderates anxiety and restores self-control.

Redirecting Attention

Another powerful tool for reducing anxiety is redirecting attention and energy. If the individual's mind is stuck thinking about a problem or worry, then it is helpful to change the direction of his or her thinking. Several strategies will help redirect thinking. Each individual must experiment to see which strategy works best: (1) direct thoughts onto the action and events around one, (2) think ahead to something enjoyable, (3) imagine oneself in a peaceful, comfortable place, or (4) deliberately absorb oneself in current activities.

Thought Stopping

Many anxiety patients report that they "can't stop" their anxious thoughts. This is especially true for persons with obsessive-compulsive disorder. Thought stopping is a behavioral technique to disrupt strong anxious thoughts.

Instruction: Place a thick rubber band around your wrist and wear that band regularly. When you notice that you are absorbed in worries, snap that rubber band. Say to yourself: "STOP IT NOW, JOE. LET IT GO." Remind yourself that the worries are part of your illness—your anxiety disorder. Once you have disrupted your thoughts, redirect your attention as described previously. Don't be discouraged if you must repeat the thought stopping several times. Repetition is necessary when anxieties and worries are strong.

Combining Relaxation Skills, Cognitive Tools, and Behavioral Change

The primary goal in treatment for anxiety disorders is for the patient to resume as normal and full an everyday lifestyle as possible, unhampered by fears and avoidance behavior. When relaxation skills and cognitive interventions are successful in reducing physiological and subjective anxiety, then these tools should be applied to assist in behavioral change. An anxious individual can employ calming and self-coaching skills to enable a return to once avoided situations and a resumption of once avoided behaviors. This return to forbidden territory, on a repeated basis, accomplishes an increasingly complete desensitization of an individual's anxiety response. In turn, the sense of self-efficacy increases further, accomplishing a more complete recovery.

As anxiety loses its grip, surprising improvements occur spontaneously, with a return to normal personal growth and motivations. As anxiety recedes, many persons report an increase in empathy with others, a renewal of feelings of fellowship and community, a return of lost aspirations and interests, and an increase in spiritual awareness.

Pharmacotherapy

Medication therapy is an adjunctive treatment that is helpful for many patients with anxiety disorders. There are several cautions in the use of antianxiety medications, however. Medication is most helpful for an individual who is also making behavioral and cognitive changes, and learning new voluntary control skills at the same time, to minimize vulnerability to future anxiety. For this reason, many physicians prefer to prescribe antianxiety medications only for those individuals who also commit to work with a cognitive-behavioral therapist, to carry out a program of skill mastery and behavioral change. This is especially true whenever avoidance behavior is part of the anxiety syndrome. The individual needs to learn to enter, confront, and master feared situations, to maintain long-term psychological health.

The medications useful for anxiety vary with the individual anxiety disorder. The benzodiazepine category of anxiolytic (antianxiety) medications is widely used for panic disorder and agoraphobia. The benzodiazepine alprazolam (Xanax®) is most widely used for panic disorder, although many practitioners are concerned about the difficulty that patients have in discontinuing alprazolam. For this reason, physicians may choose such longer-acting benzodiazepines as lorazepam (Ativan®), which is generally less habit-forming. The concern about medication dependency is greatest for individuals who have a history of alcoholism or drug dependence.

Buspiron (Buspar®) is a nonbenzodiazepine anxiolytic, widely utilized for generalized anxiety disorder. Buspar is a fairly gentle medication, less habit-forming than the benzodiazepines. It reduces an individual's ongoing level of tension and improves many patients' ability to tolerate frustration without becoming anxious or irritable. Buspar has little benefit for those with panic disorder. Venlafaxine-XR (Effexor®) is an antidepressant, which has also recently been given FDA approval for use in generalized anxiety disorder.

The selective serotonin reuptake inhibitors, or SSRIs (Luvox®, Prozac®, Zoloft®, Paxil®, Celexa®), were released as antidepressants, but at higher doses they are effective in obsessive-compulsive disorder (OCD). Many patients who were crippled by their obsessions and compulsions in past years are now able to live normal lives on the SSRIs. The SSRIs are increasingly used also in the treatment of panic disorder, agoraphobia, and social phobia. They are slow-acting medications that require at least several days and usually a month to accumulate in the bloodstream and reach their full therapeutic effect. For this reason, they cannot be taken to abort an anxiety episode. However, they are useful in reducing the frequency and intensity of anxiety episodes. As additional clinical trials are carried out with these medications, the FDA is gradually giving its approval to their extended use with the anxiety disorders. Recently, sertraline (Zoloft) and paroxetine (Paxil) were approved for use with social phobia, and sertraline was also approved for use with posttraumatic stress disorder.

Beta-blocking medications, such as the antihypertensive medication propranolol (Inderal®), atenolol (Tenormin®), and timolol maleate (Blocadren®), have also used widely for the social anxieties, and especially for performance anxiety. These medications block the autonomic physical symptoms that accompany social anxiety: blushing, sweating, trembling, and rapid heart rate. Because the socially anxious patient becomes self-conscious about blushing and other symptoms being visible to others, the pharmacological control of these symptoms makes social and performance situations less terrifying. However, the beta-blockers have only a momentary effect and do not bring about any long-term reduction in social anxiety.

Another category of medications, the monoamine oxidase inhibitors (MAO inhibitors), which includes tranylcypromine (Parnate®) and phenelzine (Nardil®), provides fairly effective relief from social phobia, but with caveats. Patients must adhere to a rigorous restrictive diet or risk life-threatening adverse effects. Patients treated with the MAO inhibitors for social anxiety show a more rapid response than those treated solely with cognitive-behavioral therapies. There is also a higher rate of relapse, however, if medication treatment is discontinued.

The simple phobias are better treated by cognitive-behavioral therapy, alone; medication appears to offer little to no treatment for these problems. The patient should construct a behavioral hierarchy and begin to increase contact with the feared object to desensitize his or her fears. Cognitive-behavioral therapy is also preferable, in most cases, for patients with adjustment disorders. It is better to directly confront one's life problems, solve those problems that can be solved, and reach acceptance for situations beyond one's control, than to simply medicate away one's reactions to reality-based problems.

Selecting medication for posttraumatic stress disorder (PTSD) is a challenging task. First, many patients experience serious clinical depression and anxiety symptoms as their PTSD condition progresses. Antidepressant medicines (including sertraline) and antianxiety medications such as the benzodiazepines can reduce the symptoms that accompany the reliving of past traumas. Another category of medication, which is more widely known for mood leveling and as anticonvulsants, may reduce the intensely labile mood, flashbacks, and intense reliving of trauma. These medications operate as "anti-kindling agents," modulating the neurophysiological flash fire accompanying traumatic memory. Just as water on firewood moderates the process of kindling a fire, these medications reduce the sudden upsurge of intense anxiety, mood, even terror. Commonly used agents include the mood leveler lithium carbonate, and the anticonvulsants divalproex (Depakote®), gabapentin (Neurontin®), and carbamazepine (Tegretol®).

Social Phobia

The preceding discussion of strategies to manage anxiety has introduced tools useful for a variety of anxiety disorders and symptoms. As mentioned, however, anxiety disorders don't all occur in the same fashion, and they respond differently to intervention. The following is a discussion of some of the unique features of social anxiety, followed by a number of strategies specifically useful for social anxiety.

Understanding Social Phobia

Research suggests that genetics, socialization, and cognitive biases all play a clear role in the onset and continuation of social anxiety. At least one large study of twins documents that genetic vulnerability contributes to the incidence of social phobia (Kendler, Neale, Kessler, Heath, & Eaves, 1992). Family studies also show that individuals with social phobia are more likely to have first-degree relatives with social phobia than with panic disorder or simple phobia (Fyer, Mannuza, Chapman, Martin, & Klein, 1995).

Family environment and early bonding play a significant role in social anxiety (Beidel & Turner, 1998). Many parents of socially anxious children are themselves shy and socially inhibited. These parents provide less modeling of social engagement and give their children less direct instruction in how to engage with others socially. Shy mothers often shelter their children from group activities, denying them the opportunity to learn social and interpersonal skills. Fathers engage in less rough and tumble or roughhousing behavior with these children.

Children who experience secure infant-parent attachment are more likely to join social groups and establish healthy peer relationships. Maternal warmth and maternal engagement with her child also predicts the child's ability to reach out and connect with peers and peer groups (Beidel & Turner, 1998). Conversely anxious parents are more likely to produce offspring with anxiety disorders (Beidel & Turner, 1997).

More than 13% of the population meets the diagnostic criteria for social phobia at some point in their lives (Kessler et al., 1994). Children who show early socially anxiety often remain more shy, threat-sensitive, and isolated throughout childhood and adult life. They are at risk for chronic depression, anxiety, and loneliness, and often sacrifice pursuing educational and career goals to shelter themselves from social exposure. The amount of needless personal suffering and lost productivity is difficult to measure (Rapee & Heimberg, 1997; Wittchen & Beloch, 1996; Zimbardo, 1977).

Cognitive psychology has produced a large body of research investigations showing how an individual's thoughts and interpretations of the world trigger or escalate anxiety states (Beck & Emery, 1985; Halford & Foddy, 1982; Rapee & Heimberg, 1997). A socially fearful individual carries a mental "schemata" or map of the world that portrays other persons as in some way menacing and him- or herself as socially inadequate. The socially anxious individual will enter any social situation with a number of specific fears: "Will I do or say something embarrassing?" "Will my mind go blank?" "Will I be unable to continue talking?" "Will I not make sense to those around me?" "Will I tremble, shake, and show signs of my anxiety?" "Will others watch me and see that I am inadequate?" "Will others see that I am anxious, and will my troubles become public?"

One result is an inability to listen in social settings. Socially anxious individuals are typically too busy with their own anxious thoughts about a situation to effectively tune in and hear others. Those who are socially anxious engage in much thinking about others' perceptions of themselves. They spend time mentally rehearsing a "perfect" response to the other person and, consequently, don't hear much of what the other is saying.

Most socially anxious adults were also shy children who withdrew from social situations. As a result, they show many deficits in social skills, which further hampers recovery from their social anxiety. Even if one intervenes to reduce anxiety, these individuals often do not know how to initiate and maintain conversations or how to perceive and interpret social cues. Socially anxious individuals also don't understand how to select or create the setting for "normal" conversation and show an inability to initiate and plan social activities.

Socially anxious individuals appear to be vigilantly attuned to potential social threats. When presented experimentally with threat-relevant and nonthreat-relevant material, they show an attention bias: They consistently give more attention to the threatening material. They also tend to interpret ambiguous information as threatening. Once they have perceived threat, the same socially anxious individuals tend to avoid processing and recall of information relevant to social threats. Researchers have developed a "two-stage vigilance-avoidance" model to understand the response of anxious individuals to new situations. Amir and colleagues suggest that social phobics display an "automatic hypervigilance" for social threats, and then quickly implement a variety of control and avoidance strategies to avoid processing information about the threatening situations (Amir, Foa, & Coles, 2000).

The second stage of cognitive avoidance plays a critical role in the chronicity of anxiety disorders. Because an anxious individual avoids processing information about social threats, the normal processes of habituation or objective evaluation do not come into play. They don't "get used to," become comfortable with, or achieve a better understanding of social situations. The threatening aspects of a situation remain threatening and the individual, therefore, continues to engage in behavioral avoidance as well as cognitive avoidance (Amir, et al., 2000; Eckman & Shean, 1997; Mogg, Bradley, Bono, & Painter, 1997).

Foa, Franklin, Perry, and Herbert (1996) investigated critical differences in the thinking of socially anxious individuals. Their data show that socially anxious individuals are able to estimate about as accurately as other persons how likely it is that certain threatening social situations will arise. However, the socially anxious individuals overestimated the amount of suffering and distress that such social situations would cause them. After cognitive behavioral therapy, however, these individuals were better able to project a realistic estimation of the outcomes of social situations.

Socially anxious individuals display the psychophysiology and psychology of embarrassment. The common symptoms of social anxiety are mediated by the beta-adrenergic system within the autonomic nervous system; symptoms include: heart palpitations, shaking, trembling, sweating, and blushing (Beidel & Turner, 1998). The symptoms mirror an anxious self-consciousness about social exposure, and the visibility of the autonomic symptoms renders the individual more self-conscious. Once embarrassed, socially anxious individuals also underestimate how well they are performing in a social setting (Edelmann, 1985). Physiological arousal usually commences as soon as a socially anxious person begins to anticipate entering a social situation. In most cases the physiological arousal persists until the individual leaves the social setting.

Finally, it is helpful to differentiate individuals with social phobia into two subgroups (Turner et al., 1992). Those with generalized social phobia are anxious in a variety of social situations, often including both performance situations and common social engagements. They also avoid a wide variety of social situations. They are likely to display a generalized shyness and often lack basic social skills. Persons with specific social phobias are fearful in only one social situation or in a narrow range of social situations. In many cases the fears focus on such challenges as public speaking or stage performances. The individual with specific social phobia is more likely to function adequately in other social settings and to display better-developed social skills.

Individuals in the generalized social phobia group are typically more disabled by their anxiety in career, relationships, and everyday life. There is considerable overlap between this group and avoidant personality disorder (Turner et al., 1991; Widiger, 1992).

Avoid Confusing Personality Disorders with Social Phobia

The overlap between social phobia and avoidant personality disorder brings up the general question of personality disorders. It is important to understand personality disorders, if one wishes to help socially anxious individuals. When personality traits become extreme, and especially when they begin to block healthy everyday functioning, psychiatry labels them as "personality disorders." A personality disorder involves a relatively rigid, enduring, and monotonous pattern of response to a variety of situations. The individual is no longer capable of varying his or her response to what each new situation calls for. In other words, the shy individual may show some fearfulness and social uneasiness with new situations and unfamiliar persons, but the individual with a "paranoid personality disorder" will show suspicion and mistrust, regardless of the situation. For such an individual, all social situations present the threat that someone is against one and will seek to harm one!

Worse, many of the behavioral strategies for helping a socially anxious person will fail with an individual plagued with a personality disorder. The lack of progress with standard therapies is often the first clue that a personality disorder or serious psychiatric problem is present. Many features of the personality disorders will persist life-long, in spite of intervention.

Theodore Millon and Roger Davis have written the best text available on personality disorders (Millon & Davis, 1996). They identify several personality disorders that seriously disturb interpersonal relationships and contribute to social isolation: the avoidant, schizoid, paranoid, and schizotypal personality disorders. Each of these personality disorders blocks fully rewarding interaction and intimacy with others. The individual with an avoidant personality disorder desires closeness and involvement with others, but fails to reach out or actively withdraws due to fears of rejection and hurt. The lack of intimacy in this case is defensive, and the individual may be open to overtures by others offering warmth and acceptance. The schizoid individual feels little interest in close involvement with others. There is a primary detachment from relatedness, and the entire life unfolds in an asocial manner. The paranoid individual perceives others as hostile adversaries, who may deliberately harm one at any moment. He or she will vigilantly and suspiciously watch others and interpret their actions as signs of "what they are really up to." The schizotypal individual is an eccentric individual, who displays oddities in behavior and thinking that isolates him or her from others. The schizotypal person often displays delusional misinterpretations of social interactions, but the individual's behaviors and symptoms are not severe enough for a diagnosis of the mental illness of schizophrenia.

Personality disorders are chronic conditions, with fairly poor prognoses for change. Individuals with "avoidant personalities" may respond to supportive treatment and learn to overcome their fears of reaching out. However, the schizoid, paranoid, and schizotypal individuals usually require specialized psychiatric treatment and, even with such treatment, may show little change. A health professional will only create frustration if the presence of a personality disorder is overlooked and the client develops unrealistic hopes for change.

Practical Interventions for Social Anxiety and Social Phobia

The primary strategy in helping socially anxious individuals parallels the approach to other anxiety disorders. The professional will introduce: (1) cognitive restructuring skills to reduce distortions in social perceptions and expectations; (2) social skills to enable the individual to reach out, engage in conversation, and manage a normal social interaction; (3) self-control skills to reduce anxiety, including relaxation skills and self-coaching skills to reduce and manage physiological arousal; (4) behavioral modification, including exposure to social settings; and (5) medications to reduce the physiological response to social situations.

Once skills are mastered, an individual will be ready to enter social situations, engage in interactions, and overcome the social fears, inadequacy feelings, and feelings of awkwardness that emerge. The process is twofold: (1) desensitizing the anxieties that have been conditioned by years of anxiety episodes in social settings, and (2) installing confidence and mastery feelings by repeated experiences of success in social interactions.

Cognitive Restructuring

Cognitive therapy begins by educating the patient about the cognitive distortions common to all anxiety disorders, such as "all or nothing thinking," overgeneralizing, mental filtering, and others, identified by David Barlow (1994), Aaron Beck (Beck & Emery, 1985), and others. The patient learns to examine his or her own anxious thoughts, identify typical and recurrent distortions, and correct these distortions. Next, cognitive therapy identifies and confronts specific fears that inhibit the individual from entering social settings. Examples of specific social fears include: "I'll just say something stupid and feel foolish," "I can never learn to socialize, so why try," or "Everyone will notice I'm sweating and blushing, and then I'll be more alone than ever."

Cognitive therapy also confronts the typical cognitive patterns discussed previously: the vigilance for threat in social settings and the exaggerated expectation that one will be harmed by social interactions. The therapist discusses typical negative or exaggerated expectations and models disputing and modifying such expectations. Over time, the patient is encouraged to reduce vigilance for threats in each new social setting and to reassure him- or herself that social settings have typically been neutral or enjoyable. The individual can redirect attention away from possible threats and toward strategies for coping and mastery in social settings.

A patient should be encouraged to identify negative expectations as they arise, to check them out by observing social interactions, and, wherever possible, to begin substituting neutral or positive expectations for the skeptical viewpoints. In many cases an individual can formulate believable self-statements predicting increased personal mastery in social situations. Examples would be: "I'm learning how to talk with people in the church setting, and it goes better almost every single Sunday," or "my coworkers who go bowling really seem to want me to join them, and they have been nice to me every time I've gone."

Confronting Cognitive Avoidance

Cognitive therapy can guide socially anxious individuals to recognize and overcome the cognitive avoidance discussed earlier. Once he or she tunes in to possible threat in a social situation, the individual often will stop thinking about that situation, and never reevaluate the realistic risk of harm. The cognitive avoidance is accompanied by behavioral avoidance of the situation, so that the individual never behaviorally masters the perceived threat. The individual can learn to identify this mental and behavioral avoidance as it emerges and begin to deliberately rethink each situation, assessing the objective risk and the coping tools one might apply to handle the situation.

Self-Disclosure of Social Anxiety

Self-disclosure is also a helpful strategy for many socially anxious individuals. Once an individual discloses his or her social fears and self-consciousness to a safe group of accepting friends or coworkers, there is a dramatic reduction in the fear that others will notice one's anxiety. Many individuals find that they are less preoccupied with their physical symptoms after they have announced the fact of social anxiety. The disclosure makes it easier to focus on actual conversations, which improves one's listening and attunement to other persons in the social interaction.

Social Skills Training

Turner, Beidel, & Cooley (1994) have produced a helpful handbook for social effectiveness therapy. Their structured program guides a socially anxious individual through three stages of social learning: (1) social environment awareness, which includes recognition of when, where, and why to initiate and terminate interpersonal encounters; (2) interpersonal skills enhancement, which includes basic listening skills and other mechanics of successful conversations and interactions; and (3) presentation skills enhancement, which includes the skills necessary to prepare, organize, and deliver a speech or presentation. Turner et al.'s handbook provides detailed instructions for a 16-week program to enhance social effectiveness. Specific skills that can be beneficial for social phobics include:

Initiating conversations	Assertiveness skills
Maintaining conversations	Assertiveness skills (with authorities)
Attending & remembering information	Constructing the body of a speech

Effectively beginning a speech   Establishing friendships
Effectively ending a speech   Maintaining friendships
Informal presentations   Heterosexual interactions
(Beidel & Turner, 1998, p. 201)

The social effectiveness therapy model draws on proven principles of learning. First the therapist explains and models a new social skill, then the patient engages in behavioral rehearsals of the social skill, Then the therapist provides corrective feedback for any maladaptive components in the patient's new social behavior, and finally the therapist seeks opportunities to positively reinforce the new social behaviors (Turner et al., 1994).

Many socially anxious individuals have benefited from Toastmasters International, a self-help group explicitly dedicated to assisting individuals in public speaking. Although public speaking is only part of the difficulty facing individuals with generalized social phobia, Toastmasters groups have assisted many individuals with other aspects of their social fears as well. In many Toastmasters groups socially anxious individuals make up a majority or at least a significant subgroup of attendees, and the encounter with other individuals struggling with similar fears and challenges is, in itself, therapeutic and normalizing. Many social phobics are enormously relieved that they are not alone in the universe with their social fears and their difficulties in social engagements. Committing oneself to attend a regular Toastmasters meeting, interacting on a repeated basis with other group members, and speaking on both a prepared and spontaneous basis before this small group of individuals, can be an excellent supplement to formal cognitive-behavioral treatment.

However, Toastmasters groups are not always convenient or appropriate for everyone, especially if an individual is not receiving cognitive-behavioral treatment elsewhere or does not understand the bases of his or her fears. Furthermore, the levels of the groups differ and, more importantly, trained professionals do not lead them. Consequently, the cognitive and physiological aspects of performance anxiety and other social fears are not directly addressed.

Classes or workshops similar to the one described in this book offer the same exposure and support in a smaller, more structured setting under the guidance of a licensed speech-language pathologist or other professional knowledgeable about the management of social fears and communication skills. This program can be duplicated in schools and universities and provides a real service for clinicians by leading them to broaden their skills by learning how to recognize and manage anxiety.

Self-Control Skills

Biofeedback can increase the socially anxious individual's ability to relax autonomic arousal (McKinney & Gatchel, 1982). Feedback of heart rate, respiration, electrodermal response, and blood pressure can provide an individual with reliable indices of autonomic nervous system arousal. These feedback modalities can be used to guide a socially anxious individual to learn autonomic control and improve the individual's sense of confidence and control in social situations.

Most forms of relaxation training can be helpful in reducing overall fearfulness and reversing physiologic activation. Diaphragmatic breathing and autogenic training reduce general anxiety and lower autonomic nervous arousal. Meditation and imagery exercises increase an individual's control over where he or she directs attention in any situation.

Behavior Modification/Exposure Therapy

The primary goal of behavior modification in all anxiety disorders is to identify, confront, and overcome avoidance behaviors. In the case of social phobia, a patient constructs a hierarchy of social situations that provoke anxiety and avoidance, ranking experiences from least frightening to most frightening (See Figure 5-4). Next the patient begins to imagine entering, desensitizing, and mastering situations low in the hierarchy and proceeds up the hierarchy through his or her imagination. The individual visualizes confronting each situation until the imaginary exposure becomes comfortable at each level and then proceeds higher up the hierarchy. Actual exposure in situ in social settings follows, with the patient drawing on self-talk, self-reassurance, new social skills, and self-quieting skills to ease the discomfort of each new social situation, until he or she becomes comfortable in that new situation.

Medication

As mentioned in the section on pharmacotherapy, medications such as the antihypertensive medication propranolol are beta-blockers and prevent the onset of the autonomic symptoms mentioned in that discussion. The medication enables an individual to feel less scrutinized by those provoking anxiety and, thus, reduces self-consciousness. Antidepressant medications, especially the SSRIs, reduce vulnerability to social anxiety and often increase an individual's confidence in entering social situations. MAO inhibitors given for social anxiety lead to a more rapid response than treatment solely with cognitive-behavioral therapies. Yet, there are serious medical cautions and a higher rate of relapse, if MAO treatment is discontinued.

Chapter Summary

This chapter has highlighted the importance of identifying anxiety disorders. Speech-language pathologists (SLPs) will greatly enhance their professional skills if they routinely screen for and recognize the signs of anxiety, use the listed screening questions, and communicate to clients about the probability of an anxiety disorder and the availability of effective professional help. In the course of providing speech-language therapy, SLPs can also teach some self-regulation skills, which may be sufficient to help a mildly to moderately anxious individual to manage his or her anxiety. Relaxation skills and cognitive self-help skills, such as floating, thought-stopping, and redirecting attention, can help many individuals to manage their anxiety symptoms that may be contributing to or exacerbating their presenting communication disorders and help them to maintain a more active and fulfilling life.

If a clinician is unable to help the clients with an anxiety disorder, they can provide a great service to the patient or client by explaining the problem and referring him or her to appropriate mental health professionals. Similarly, teachers, trainers, and other communication specialists who are interested in offering services to overcome communication apprehension and performance anxiety must also understand the nature of anxiety and its management and incorporate this information into their curricula.

Remember that socially anxious individuals will be doubly self-conscious about any obvious speech or voice problem and will probably make even more rapid improvement if their inordinate anxiety is addressed. If anxiety continues to disrupt an individual's everyday life or interferes with the client's therapeutic progress, he or she should be referred to a cognitive-behavioral therapist who is experienced and skilled in treating the anxiety disorders.

Clients need to hear the message: "I see several signs here of an anxiety disorder. Many people suffer similar anxiety; you are not alone. Help is available, and most people can recover completely. I can teach you a few skills that will help you to manage your anxiety. If that isn't enough help, I can give you the names of some effective therapists who will help you to control your anxiety."

References

Adams-Webber, J. & Mancuso, J. C. (Eds.). (1983). *Applications of personal construct theory*. New York: Academic Press.

American Psychiatric Association. (1994). *The diagnostic and statistical manual of mental disorders, fourth edition (DSM-IV)*. Washington, DC: The American Psychiatric Association.

Amir, N., Foa, E.B. & Coles, M.E. (2000). Implicit memory bias for threat-relevant information in individuals with generalized social phobia. *Journal of Abnormal Psychology, 109 (4)*, 713-720.

Bandura, A. (1997). *Self-efficacy: The exercise of control*. New York: W.H. Freeman.

Barlow, D. H. (Ed.). (1994. *Clinical handbook of psychological disorders: A step-by-step treatment manual*. New York: Guilford.

Beck, A. T. & Emery, G. (1985). *Anxiety disorders and phobias*. New York: Basic Books.

Beidel, D. C. & Turner, S. M. (1997). At risk for anxiety: I. Psychopathology in the offspring of anxious parents. *Journal of the Academy of Child and Adolescent Psychiatry, 36*, 918–924.

Beidel, D. C. & Turner, S. M. (1998). *Shy children, phobic adults*. Washington, DC: American Psychological Association.

Beidel D. C., Turner, S. M., & Dancu, C. V. (1985). Physiological, cognitive and behavioral aspects of social anxiety. *Behavior Research and Therapy, 23*, 109–117.

Benson, H. (1975). *The relaxation response*. New York: Morrow.

Conway, A. (1994). Breathing and feeling: Capnography and the individually meaningful stressor. *Biofeedback and Self-Regulation, 19*, 135–139.

Coryell, W. & Winokur, G. (Eds.). (1991). *The clinical management of anxiety disorders*. New York: Oxford University Press.

Curran, J. P., Wallander, J. L., & Fischetti, M. (1980). The importance of behavioral and cognitive factors in heterosexual-social anxiety. *Journal of Personality, 48*, 285–292.

Eckman, P. S. & Shean, G. D. (1997). Habituation of cognitive and physiological arousal and social anxiety. B*ehavior Research and Therapy, 35*,1113–1121.

Edelmann, R. J. (1985). Dealing with embarrassing events: Socially anxious and non-socially anxious groups compared. *British Journal of Clinical Psychology, 24* (Pt 4), 281–288.

Emmelkamp, P. M. G., Bouman, T. K., & Scholing, A. (1992). *Anxiety disorders: A practitioner's guide*. Chichester, England: John Wiley and Sons.

Everly, G. S. (1989). *A clinical guide to the treatment of the human stress response*. New York: Plenum.

Fischer, W. F. (1970). *Theories of anxiety*. New York: Harper & Row.

Foa, E. B., Franklin, M. E., Perry, K. J., & Herbert, J. D. (1996). Cognitive biases in generalized social phobia. *Journal of Abnormal Psychology, 105*, 433–439.

Foa, E. B. & Kozak, M. L. (1998). Clinical applications of bioinformational theory: Understanding anxiety and its treatment. *Behavior Therapy, 29*, 675–690.

Fyer, A. J., Mannuza, S., Chapman, T. F., Martin, L. Y., & Klein, D. F. (1995). Specificity in family aggregation of phobic disorders. *Archives of General Psychiatry, 52*, 564–573.

Gold, M. S. (1989). *The good news about panic, anxiety, and phobias*. New York: Villard Books.

Greist, J. H. & Jefferson, J. W. (Eds.). (1995). *Obsessive-compulsive disorders casebook*. Washington, DC: American Psychiatric Press.

Halford, K. & Foddy, M. (1982). Cognitive and social skills correlates of social anxiety. *British Journal of Clinical Psychology, 21,*17–28.

Holt, C. S., Heimberg, R. G., & Hope, D. A. (1992). Avoidant personality disorder and the generalized subtype of social phobia. *Journal of Abnormal Psychology, 101*, 318–325.

Kelly, G. A. (1955). *The psychology of personal constructs* (vols. 1 & 2). New York: Norton. [Second edition 1991, London/New York: Routledge and the Centre for Personal Construct Psychology/]

Kelly, G. A. (1963). A theory of personality: The psychology of personal constructs. New York: W. W. Norton.

Kendler, K. S., Neale, M. C., Kessler, R. C., Heath, A. C., & Eaves, L. J. (1992). The genetic epidemiology of social phobia in women: The relationship of agoraphobia, social phobia, situational phobia, and simple phobia. *Archives of General Psychiatry, 49*, 273–281.

Kessler, R. C., McGonagle, K. A., Zhao, S., Nelson, C. B., Hughes, M., Eshelman, S., Wittchen, H., & Kendler, K. S. (1994). Lifetime and 12-month prevalence of DSM-III-R psychiatric disorders in the United States. *Archives of General Psychiatry, 51*, 8–19.

Knapp, S. & VandeCreek, L. (1994). *Anxiety disorders: A scientific approach for selecting the most effective treatment*. Sarasota, FL: Professional Resources Press.

Linder, L. M. & Der-Karabetian, A. (1986). Social anxiety, public self-consciousness, and variability of behavior. *Psychological Reports, 59,* 206.

McKinney M. E. & Gatchel, R. J. (1982). The comparative effectiveness of heart rate biofeedback, speech skills training, and a combination of both in treating public-speaking anxiety. *Biofeedback and Self Regulation, 7, 71–87.*

Millon, T. & Davis, R. D. (1996). *Disorders of personality: DSM-IV and beyond.* New York: John Wiley and Sons.

Mogg, K., Bradley, B. P., Bono, J. D., & Painter, M. (1997). Time course of attentional bias for threat information in non-clinical anxiety. *Behavior Research and Therapy, 35,* 297–303.

Pervin, L. A. (1975). *Personality: Theory, assessment, and research.* New York: Wiley.

Rachman, S. (1982). Fear and courage: Some military aspects. *Journal of the Royal Army Medical Corps, 128,* 100–104 .

Rachman, D. (1999, April). *Fear and courage.* Keynote address to the annual meeting of the Association for Applied Psychophysiology and Biofeedback, Vancouver, British Columbia.

Rapee, R. M. & Heimberg, R. G. (1997). A cognitive-behavioral model of anxiety in social phobia. *Behavior Research and Therapy, 35,* 741–756.

Regier, D. A., Narrow, W. E., & Rae, D. S. (1990). The epidemiology of anxiety disorders. The epidemiological catchment area (ECA) experience. *Journal of Psychiatric Research, 24*(2), 9–14.

Sheehan, D. V. (1983). *The anxiety disease.* New York: Scribners.

Stein, M. B., Baird, A., & Walker, J. R. (1996). Social phobia in adults with stuttering. *American Journal of Psychiatry, 153,* 278–280.

Stemberger, R. T., Turner, S. M., Beidel, D. C., & Calhoun, K. S. (1995). Social phobia: An analysis of possible developmental factors. *Journal of Abnormal Psychology, 104,* 526–531.

Timmons, B., & Ley, R. (1994). *Behavioral and psychological approaches to breathing disorders.* New York: Plenum.

Turner, S. M., Beidel, D. C., Borden, J. W., Stanley, M. A., & Jacob, R. G. (1991). Social phobia: Axis I and II correlates. *Journal of Abnormal Psychology, 100,* 102–106.

Turner, S. M., Beidel, D. C., & Cooley, M.R. (1994). *Social effectiveness therapy: A program for overcoming social anxiety and social phobia.* Charleston, SC: Turndel Publishing.

Turner, S. M., Beidel, D. C., & Townsley, R. M. (1992). Social phobia: A comparison of specific and generalized subtypes and avoidant personality disorder. *Journal of Abnormal Psychology, 101,* 326–331.

van der Kolk, B. A. (Ed.). (1987). *Psychological trauma.* Washington, DC: American Psychiatric Press, Inc.

van der Kolk, B. A. & Greenberg, M. S. (1987). The psychobiology of the trauma response: Hyperarousal, constriction, and addiction to traumatic reexposure. In B. A. van der Kolk (Ed.), *Psychological trauma* (pp. 63–87). Washington, DC: American Psychiatric Press, Inc.

Weeks, C. (1978). *Peace from nervous suffering.* New York: Bantam Books.

Widiger, T. A. (1992). Generalized social phobia versus avoidant personality disorder: A commentary on three studies. *Journal of Abnormal Psychology, 101,* 340–343.

Wittchen, H. U. & Beloch, E. (1996). The impact of social phobia on quality of life. *International Clinics in Psychopharmacology, 11*(3), 15–23.

Zimbardo, P. (1977). *Shyness: What it is, what to do about it.* Reading, MA: Addison-Wesley.

CHAPTER

4

Physiological Perspectives

The Physiology of Stress[†]

Richard Gevirtz, Ph.D.[*]

Part I: Physiological Response to Stress

The Transactional Model of Stress

Modern definitions of "stress" are primarily based on the transactional model originally described by Lazarus and Folkman (1984). In essence "potentially stressful events are appraised as either stressful or benign in the context of an individual's own values, beliefs experiences, and coping resources" (Cohen, 1992, p. 110).

With this general model in mind, this chapter describes basic concepts and some recent developments in the physiology and biology of stress. Because this is an enormous topic, I will focus primarily on the

[†] Originally published as "The Physiology of Stress," by R. Gevirtz, in *Stress and Health Research and Clinical Applications*, (pp. 53–72), J. G. Carlson, F. J. McGuigan, and J. L. Sheppard (Eds.), Amsterdam, The Netherlands: Harwood Academic Publishers, © 2000 OPA (Oversees Publishers Association) N.V. with permission from Gordon and Breach Publishers.

[*]Dr. Richard Gevirtz is a professor in the Health Psychology Program at the California School of Professional Psychology (CSPP) in San Diego. He has been involved in research and clinical work in applied psychophysiology for the last 25 years. His primary interests are in understanding the physiological and psychological mediators involved in disorders such as chronic muscle pain, panic disorder, fibromyalgia, chronic fatigue syndrome, gastrointestinal pain, functional cardiac disorder, etc. He is the author of many journal articles and chapters on these topics.

autonomic nervous system and secondarily on the endocrine system/immune systems.

It is useful to conceive of the stress response as one that has evolved in humans in a highly social context. Our perception of acceptance or rejection in our social interactions determines a good deal of what is meant by stress in an everyday context. This is a bit of a departure from earlier works (e.g., Selye, 1956)[1] that emphasized the role of the endocrine response in much more primitive and directly life-threatening situations and interpolated findings from these extreme settings to "everyday" stressors. Thus, endocrine and pituitary medullary responses to parachute jumping (Ursin, Baade, & Levine, 1978) were thought to constitute a model for all stressors, rather than for only dramatically threatening events. Modern conceptualizations have made this distinction and have emphasized the more transient and responsive autonomic systems. Endocrine-based measures may not be sufficiently sensitive to measure the effects of daily stressors and hassles (e.g., Cummins & Gevirtz, 1992), whereas autonomic measures contain a wealth of information for these more common stressors.

The Autonomic Nervous System

Guyton and Hall (1995) offer an excellent overview of the medical physiology in the major stress systems. Guyton (1976) provides more detailed coverage. The nervous system is divided into two main divisions: the central nervous system (CNS), consisting of the brain and spinal cord, and the peripheral nervous system, consisting of the somatic/sensory system and the autonomic nervous system (ANS). The ANS has two branches: the sympathetic (SNS) and the parasympathetic (PNS). Most traditional work has centered on the ANS for understanding the physiology of stress. The ANS functions with visceral and other organ systems in the body. In many systems, it functions as the sole regulatory pathway, Although in others it shares regulatory functions with other systems. The ANS is activated mainly by centers in the spinal cord, the hypothalamus, and the brainstem. Although these centers are important, it is worth noting that the cerebral cortex can also exert an influence. Recent work on developmental psychobiology has revealed fascinating relationships between late-developing brain centers, such as

---

[1] Contemporary notions of the relationship between stress and health began with this Canadian endocrinologist. Selye said stress can be as harmful to health as disease and noted individual differences in people's ability to cope with stessors, based on attitudes, perceptions, beliefs, and copy strategies, as well as genetic and acquired physiological factors. (B. H.)

the orbitofrontal cortex, and the down regulation of the ANS. This material was recently compiled in a fascinating book by Allan Schore (1994).

The Sympathetic Branch

The SNS has long been thought of as the "stress nervous system," because it seems to mobilize resources in the body for emergency situations such as those requiring "fight or flight response." Although this conceptualization is generally correct, it has been shown to be too simplistic in many ways. The name, itself, implies that the system works as an orchestra, with all parts in "sympathy" to all other parts, thus creating a unified mass action response to perceived threats, physiological trauma, or other types of dysregulation. This idea is based partly on the anatomy of the system itself. The sympathetic nerves originate in the spinal column between T-1 and L-2 and travel to paravertebral sympathetic chains. From there, they travel to target organs: the heart, the bronchi,the gut, the adrenal medulla, the kidney, and other sites. In this organization, the system is unique, in that there is a distinctive preganglionic fiber to the chain and a postganglionic fiber to the target organ. By setting up this chain-like way station, communication among the elements of the system is greatly enhanced. The preganglionic fibers can synapse with the postganglionic fibers and innervate the target organs directly. They can travel up and down in the chain to influence other organs. In this way, complicated communication is possible. Many of the postganglionic fibers pass back to become spinal nerves and radiate throughout the body as skeletal nerves that can influence blood vessels, sweat glands, and piloerector muscles.

One group of preganglionic sympathetic nerves passes through the chain, through the splanchnic[2] nerves, and finally synapses at the adrenal medullae. They stimulate specialized nerve endings that secrete epinephrine (adrenaline) and norepinephrine (noradrenaline) into the circulating blood. These hormones are carried to almost all parts of the body, where they have an effect similar to the direct sympathetic innervation, except that the effect is much longer acting (up to 10 times). Thus, as various effects on target organs occur, the adrenal medullary pathway recreates almost the same response, but with a much longer duration.

The overall architecture of the SNS allows for specificity or mass action, depending on the environmental demands. The preganglionic/postganglionic split, with up and down connections, ensures this flexibility.

Neurotransmitters are the chemical communicators in the nervous system. The neurotransmitters in the sympathetic system are a bit more

---

[2] relating to the viscera

complicated than those in the other peripheral systems. In both the SNS and PNS, there are two basic synaptic transmitters: norepinephrine and acetylcholine. Fibers that secrete the former are called adrenergic, and those secreting the latter are labeled cholinergic. All preganglionic fibers (those going from the spinal cord to the paravertebral ganglionic chain) are cholinergic. This is true in both the SNS, where the distinction between pre- and postganglionic fibers is dramatic, and also in the PNS, where the postganglionic fibers are quite short and primarily located at the target organ site itself. This is the reason that any acetcholine-like substance can trigger both PNS and SNS target organs, when applied at the ganglia.

The postganglionic fibers in the PNS are all cholinergic, but in the SNS they are mostly adrenergic. The primary exceptions to this rule are the sweat glands, along with a few blood vessels, which are cholinergically innervated. Thus a great deal of pharmacological interest has centered on adrenergic blockers or, conversely, on reducing cholinergic reactions to psychoactive drugs.

Research with cholinergic and adrenergic drugs has shown that there are a variety of receptor types within both the PNS and SNS. The two main acetylcholine receptors have been classified as "muscarinic"—because they are activated by only muscarine (a poison found in toadstools)—and "nicotinic" (stimulated by nicotine only). Acetylcholine stimulates both of them. Several adrenergic receptor types have been found, and more discoveries are anticipated. These receptors have been classified as "beta" and "alpha" types. "Beta$_1$" and "beta$_2$" subtypes are firmly established. Other types have been detected, but not yet established. Both alpha and beta receptors can be excitatory or inhibitory.

Alpha receptors produce vasodilation, iris dilation, intestinal relaxation, intestinal sphincter contraction, pilomotor contraction, bladder sphincter contraction, and (recently discovered) muscle spindle activation.

Beta receptors produce vasodilation, cardioacceleration, increased myocardial strength, intestinal relaxation, bronchodilation, calorigenesis, glycogenolysis, lipolysis, and bladder relaxation. Many drugs that are agonists or antagonists of these systems exist. For example, propranolol is a well-known beta-blocker that produces a kind of "peripheral relaxation." Because of this effect, it is sometimes used by performing artists or athletes.

The organs targeted by the ANS are well known. By reviewing the major targets, the stage is set for considering what is currently known about various disorders that have been thought to be mediated by sympathetic pathways.

Table 4-1 shows the target organ and the effects of sympathetic and parasympathetic stimulation.

In addition to the direct SNS pathways to target organs, the adrenals are also recruited by the SNS by way of direct pathways to the adrenal medulla and through indirect hypothalamic-pituitary-adrenocortical pathways.

Recently, sympathetic pathways to the muscle spindle have been documented in several species. The spindle is the sensory organ for muscle, regulating length and stretch. It has also been shown to contain nociceptive afferents (Barker & Banks, 1986; Passatore, Fillipi, & Grassi, 1985). This discovery of sympathetic enervation may explain the long-observed relationship between "muscle tension" and stress. Myofascial trigger points are "hyperirritable spots, usually within a taut band of skeletal muscle or in the muscle's fascia that is painful on compression and can give rise to characteristic referred pain, tenderness, and autonomic phenomena" (Travel & Simons, 1983, p.4). I have found that these myofascial trigger points are quite responsive to stimuli thought to stimulate the SNS, and they can be blocked only by sympathetic blockers. EMG activity in the trigger point generates activity at high levels, while a needle, at the same depth in adjacent nontender muscle, is essentially quiet (Hubbard & Berkoff, 1993). It is my belief that trigger points are muscle spindles that have been overactivated by emotional stresses, physical demands on the muscle, trauma, or combinations of these factors. This discovery may open up new avenues to the study of SNS activation of target organ activity (Gevirtz, Hubbard, & Harpin, 1996; McNulty, Gevirtz, Hubbard, & Berkoff, 1994).

TABLE 4-1. Autonomic effects on various organs of the body

Organ		Effect of Sympathetic Stimulation	Effect of Parasympathetic Stimulation
Eye:	Pupil	Dilated	Constricted
	Ciliary muscle	Slight relaxation	Contracted
Glands:	Nasal	Vasoconstriction and slight secretion	Stimulation of thin, copious secretion (containing many enzymes for enzyme-secreting glands)
	Lacrimal		
	Parotid		
	Submaxillary		
	Gastric		
	Pancreatic		
Sweat Glands		Copious sweating (cholinergic)	None
Apocrine glands		Thick, odoriferous secretion	None

(continues)

TABLE 4-1. *continued*

Organ		Effect of Sympathetic Stimulation	Effect of Parasympathetic Stimulation
Heart:	Muscle	Increased rate Increased force of contraction	Slowed rate Decreased force of atrial contraction
	Coronaries	Dilated (β_2); constricted (α)	Dilated
Lungs:	Bronchi	Dilated	Constricted
	Blood vessels	Mildly constricted	? Dilated
Gut: Lumen		Decreased peristalsis and tone	Increased peristalsis and tone
Sphincter		Increased tone	Relaxed
Liver		Glucose released	Slight glycogen synthesis
Gallbladder and bile ducts		Relaxed	Contracted
Kidney		Decreased output	None
Bladder: Detrusor		Relaxed	Excited
Trigone		Excited	Relaxed
Penis		Ejaculation	Erection
Systemic blood vessels:		Constricted	None
Abdominal		Constricted (adrenergic α)	None
muscle		Dilated (adrenergic β) Dilated (cholinergic)	
	Skin	Constricted	None
Blood:	Coagulation	Increased	None
	Glucose	Increased	None
Basal metabolism		Increased up to 100%	None
Adrenal medullary secretion		Increased	None
Mental activity		Increased	None
Piloerector muscles		Excited	None
Skeletal muscle		Increased glycogenolysis Increased strength	None

Note. From *Textbook of Medical Physiology* (9th ed.) (p. 775), by A. Guyton and J. E. Hall, 1996, Philadelphia: W. B. Saunders. © 1981 by W. B. Saunders Company. Reprinted with permission.

The gastrointestinal (GI) system is heavily influenced primarily by the parasympathetic system, although it contains an intrinsic nervous system of its own, the intramural plexus. The PNS increases overall GI tract activity that involves prolonged peristalsis (kneading-like slow contractions) and sphincter relaxation. The SNS has the effect of rapidly halting GI activity by way of the greater, lesser, and least splanchnic nerves that emerge from the spinal column at T-5/T-6, T-9, and T-11, respectively.

Blood vessels in the viscera and skin are constricted by sympathetic activity but they are little affected by parasympathetic activity. One notable exception to this rule is seen in facial areas such as the cheeks, which can be dilated by PNS enervation (e.g., blushing). The work of Robert Freedman (1991; Freedman et al., 1988) has clearly demonstrated that finger blood flow is reduced under sympathetic influence. In contrast, voluntary increases, such as biofeedback-based finger temperature elevations, are mediated by blood-borne beta-adrenergic compounds. Thus, the role of the SNS in relaxation-type interventions is probably more complicated than may have been previously thought. When someone is taught to warm his or her hands (to, for example, 94°), it can be assumed that systemic factors that transcend the ANS, are at work.

Arterial blood pressure is also influenced by SNS activity in that it is the result of increased cardiac output and increased peripheral resistance. PNS pathways have a mild effect because they slow down heart rate and indirectly lower blood pressure.

In addition to these modes of control, blood pressure is also influenced by autonomic reflexes, primarily the baroreceptor reflex. Stretch receptors in the aorta and carotid arteries, when stimulated by high blood pressures, signal the brainstem, which inhibits sympathetic action and promotes parasympathetic action to the heart and blood vessels. This system is keenly sensitive to acute changes but quickly adapts to long-term levels. The baroreceptor system has an oscillating rhythm of about 10 seconds. This phenomena is called the Traube-Hering-Mayer wave. Recently, much work has centered on understanding baroreceptor sensitivity (BRS). Hypertensives, or even those with a family history of hypertension show lowered BRS than normotensives (Eckberg & Sleight, 1992). Measurement of BRS may turn out to be of interest to psychophysiological disorders because it is a sensitive indicator of ANS/PNS feedback coherence and may be affected by "stress" over time.

Dual control by the SNS and PNS is seen in the lungs, where bronchodilation is sympathetically controlled, and bronchoconstriction is parasympathetically controlled. Many more examples of this reciprocal relationship probably exist and await further research.

The Sympathetic/Adrenal Medullae

As mentioned previously, parts of the sympathetic response are backed up by a blood-borne system of hormones secreted by the core or medulla of the adrenal glands. Sympathetic stimulation causes large quantities of epinephrine and norepinephrine to be released into the bloodstream. These circulating hormones have effects on the target organs similar to those described earlier, except that the effects are of much greater duration (up to 10 times longer). The two hormones differ from each other slightly. Epinephrine produces more dramatic cardiovascular effects and greatly increases metabolism (up to 100%), with norepinephrine having a more potent effect on peripheral resistance and, therefore, blood pressure. The sympathetic/adrenal medullary system is one of many examples of redundant systems built into the body. Failure of either the SNS system at the target organs or of the adrenal medullae has little effect on the overall organism.

The Parasympathetic System (PNS)

As was mentioned earlier and shown in Table 4-1, the PNS is simpler in structure than the SNS and has always been presumed to have more organ specificity. This system is characterized as facilitating restoration and maintenance of the organism. However, withdrawal of the system during stress may also play an important role.

Most research has been aimed at the reciprocal relationship between the SNS and PNS in the functioning of the cardiac system. Porges (1995) has added much to our knowledge of the PNS with regard to conceptualizations of stress. He describes the PNS as a polyvagal system with two branches. The first, the vegetative vagal system is older in an evolutionary sense. The second, labeled the "smart vagus," originates in the nucleus ambiguous of the brainstem. The more primitive vegetative vagus acts to preserve resources, as one would expect to see in reptiles. That is, it greatly diminishes cardiac activity as exemplified in the primitive diving reflex.[3] This system is balanced by the mammalian "smart" vagus, which regulates the more social functions such as facial muscle flexibility, vocal functions, and swallowing, and also controls the respiratory modulation of the heart. These PNS pathways are often ignored in the study of stress, but may be of great importance in facial EMG studies and in understanding how social hierarchies can be stimuli for a stress response.

A respiratory oscillator in the medulla has a periodicity of about 8–12 seconds (.12 to .30 Hz) and when seen in the heart period is called respiratory sinus arrhythmia (RSA). Many observers have described the RSA system as "withdrawing" during stress. Thus, you may see vagal tone as a measure in stress studies. Psychophysiologists have been especially interested in PNS activity here because of the airway constriction occurring in asthma. Porges (1995) presents an in-depth

---

[3] The primitive diving reflex in mammals occurs when a sensory stimulus such as cold water or ice touches the face. It can prolong survival by triggering reflex inhibition of the respiratory center (apnea), bradycardia, and vasoconstriction to conserve tissue in the heart, brain, or other organs.

theoretical review of this idea, and Bernston, Cacioppo, & Quigley (1993) give a review of the physiology of this response system. By measuring the power or amplitude of frequencies around the breathing rhythm (.12 to .30 Hz), one can discern the parasympathetic or "vagal tone" influencing the heart rate. In this way, it might be possible to get a more integrated view of how the two branches of the ANS may interact to control organ systems and thus disorders of those systems.

SNS and PNS Complex Interactions

Although the SNS and PNS can be thought of as separate, like almost all aspects of the nervous system, they often work in complex interactive ways. A great deal of recent physiological research has tried to better understand these functions. For example, Bernston, Cacioppo, and Quigley (1991) have constructed "topological" maps that show how PNS/SNS reciprocity and coactivity might work at various levels of each. They advance an alternative to the "single vector model" of the autonomic continuum. Although simple linear response curves representing the relationship between psychological and physiological variables have often failed, with "independent measures of the relative activity of both ANS divisions within an organ state, or its reactive change, in the dimensions of autonomic space" (p. 482), a more complete description is possible.

It seems clear that psychophysiology will be greatly enriched by the technological advances that allow noninvasive monitoring of subtle autonomic functions. Many psychophysiological and anxiety disorders are probably associated with subtle autonomic dysfunction or the breakdown of homeostasis in the ANS. Better understanding of the nuances of ANS functioning could promote improved diagnosis and treatment.

General Considerations

An important feature of the ANS is the concept of "tone." Both the SNS and PNS maintain an adequate frequency rate to keep the target organ at a midrange value. In this way excitation or inhibition can be used for regulation. Beyond this, the two branches interact in several organ systems to further complicate the picture.

Modern research of the ANS has emphasized the complexity of the system. As an example, Jänig & McLachlan (1992) talk about "functional pathways" as the "building blocks of the autonomic nervous system." They trace the history of the ANS conceptualization from Langley to Cannon,[4] to Hess, to the present. "The idea that the sympathetic outflow

[4] In 1926 Cannon introduced the concept of homeostasis, the adaption of the body to stay in balance. Cannon wrote extensively on the ANS role in the stress response, and was also the first to develop the concept of the "fight or flight" response process (B. H.)

to the cardiovascular and visceral systems is always activated in parallel remains firmly ensconced in modern textbooks, usually contrasted with the so-called specificity of the parasympathetic system" (Jänig & McLachlan, 1992, p. 5). Actually, modern recording techniques have elucidated many very distinct systems within the SNS. Among the examples cited are distinct vasoconstrictor systems (muscle versus cutaneous) and visceral organs regulated completely independently of cardiovascular systems. Jänig and McLachlan (1992) state, "It is therefore quite clear that 'sympathetic tone,' as such, simply does not exist" (p. 8). In fact, the SNS must be studied as a complex system with differentiation throughout the peripheral and central nervous systems. Likewise, the PNS has recently been described as having distinct branches that may have evolved in mammals to better adapt to complex environmental demands (Porges, 1995). "The behavioral derivatives of the two branches of the vagus suggest a typology in which one branch of the vagus deals with unconscious reflexive vegetative function and the other is involved in more conscious, voluntary, flexible and often social activities" (p. 309). The vegetative vagus contains only visceral efferents, while the smart vagus innervates the somatic musculature of the palate, larynx, pharynx, and esophagus.

During stress, the two branches can be thought of as being in conflict, with the vegetative vagus trying to shut down the cardiovascular system (as in the diving reflex), and the smart vagus withdrawing vagal tone as an adaptation to "novelty in the environment while coping with the need to maintain metabolic output and continuous social communication" (p. 310).

This "polyvagal" model may lead us to a much richer knowledge of the relationships among the branches and among specific classes of stressors, with their distinct physiological patterns. Because the smart vagus can be seen in the light of evolutionary adaptations, it leads us to reemphasize the social context of stress.

Endocrine Stress Responses

Hans Selye (1956, 1973) has elucidated a comprehensive homeostatic model of stress, centered mostly on the endocrine response systems. With the conceptualization of the general adaptation syndrome (GAS), he postulated that the normal adaptation process maintains healthy homeostasis and enhances the organism's ability to meet threats, but that prolonged stressors would result in a physiological "exhaustion" state that would lead to organ pathology. Ulcers served as the prototypical disease for the model.

This model was formulated primarily on observations of animals in physiological labs. It had been shown that a cortical interpretation of a threat to homeostasis leads to hypothalamic activation with neural control of the posterior lobe of the pituitary gland (through corticotropin-releasing hormone [CHA]). The pituitary, in turn, releases adrenocorticotropin hormone (ACTH) into the bloodstream, where it targets the adrenal cortex. The adrenal cortex releases glucocorticoids, anti-inflammatory substances that try to control the consequences of trauma. This response is much slower and occurs in the aftermath of the initial sympathetic or even the adrenomedullary response. Selye (1936) early on had noted the nonspecificity of the pituitary-adrenocortical system. A great number of physical, chemical, and psychological stimuli seem to be able to accelerate the production of glucocorticoids by the adrenal cortex. This is unusual in biology, where specificity of innervation is the rule. This led Selye to conclude that the system evolved to be responsive to a wide variety of stressors (Saffran & Dokas, 1983). Although many other hormones are affected by stress (insulin, prolactin, thyroid hormones, epinephrine, glucagon, endorphins, and enkephalins), the adrenal hormonal response has been the major focus of research on the physiology of stress. Studies with adrenalectomized animals have shown that the heightened anxiety and stress response that occurs after surgery, can be reversed with corticosterone (a glucocorticoid; File, Vellucci, & Wendlandt, 1979).

Modern versions of the GAS emphasize the biphasic role of the adrenal steroids, first to counteract inflammation and then to set up buffers to protect tissue from their overreaction (Munck, Guyre, & Holbrook, 1984). Moreover, it is now known that stress hormones can affect virtually every organ system in the body, especially the brain (McEwen & Mendelson, 1993). The key concept here is "counterregulation." Adrenal steroids seem to play an important role in countering many of the body's initial responses to stress, maintaining a critical balance. For example, glucocorticoid helps to keep the noradrenergic arousal system in check. This may serve an antidepressive function, because it has been shown that a hyperactive or dysregulated noradrenergic system is associated with depression (Gold, Goodwin, & Chrousos, 1988). No doubt, future research will uncover many complex interactions between stress hormones and neurotransmitter systems.

Taken as a whole, it appears likely that stress hormones play an important role in depressive disease. Prolonged exposure to uncontrollable stressors seems to dysregulate seratonergic receptor sites. Benzodiazepine and seratonergic systems also seem to exhibit complex biphasic responses to stress hormones (McEwan & Mendelson, 1993). With the rapid advances in psychopharmacology, these relationships should emerge and broaden the scope of the physiology of stress.

Respiratory Response Systems

Until recently, respiratory responses were rarely mentioned in coverage of stress physiology. However, there is an extensive literature on this and related topics that goes back almost 100 years (Han et al., 1997). The basic idea in this literature is that stress, or more importantly, prolonged stress, can lead to hyperventilation (breathing at a faster rate than metabolically needed) which, by altering the acid-base balance, can lead to a constellation of symptoms such as, dyspnea, panic, fatigue, anxiety, dizziness, muscle weakness, and so on. Several recent books have emphasized the importance of such constellations in a variety of disorders (Fried, 1993; Timmons & Ley, 1994) .

To briefly summarize, it has been shown that there exists a transient response to stress, characterized by rapid, shallow, breathing that leads to a slight elevation in the acid-base balance of the body (that is, in the direction of alkalinity). Although this response seems to produce short-term anxiolytic and analgesic effects, when the response is prolonged it can lead to the symptoms described. For example, cortical blood flow is reduced, vasoconstriction can occur, the cardiovascular system is activated, muscle tone is increased, gastrointestinal disruption can occur, and the coronary artery can even become constricted.

The bases for these changes are complex and multifaceted. One important system that has been understood for many years is the oxygen dissociation curve. The oxygen dissociation curve is a well-known physiological law that shows the relationship between blood pH and the ability of oxygen to be released from hemoglobin. As blood pH becomes more alkaline, the oxygen becomes overbound to the hemoglobin molecule. This means that oxygen is not as available to organs in the body (including the cerebral cortex).[5] There is evidence (although this is controversial) that prolonged overbreathing can become homoeostatically set in such a manner as to create the symptoms described, yet allow ostensibly normal physiological function. This state of affairs has been labeled the "hyperventilation syndrome." It is a diagnostic entity that has been popular in Europe.

The Striate Musculature

The striate musculature, independent of the spindle/sympathetic interactions described earlier, does play a reactive role in the stress response. This may be seen in two ways: very short latency muscle contractions

---

[5] The lack of oxygen to the brain possibly underlies complaints of forgetfulness, word-finding difficulty, and thought organization problems of fear-ridden speakers. Slow, diaphragmatic breathing enables reversal of blood alkalinity and subsequent calming. (B. H.)

(under 100 msec) and muscle bracing or splinting. McGuigan has described these responses (1978) in various locations. It is clear from the timing sequences that a rapid muscular contraction is among the body's first responses to a stressful stimulus. Speech muscles respond to both words and letters with latencies of 44 to 85 ms (Davis, 1983). Similarly, Bickford et al.(1964) reported very rapid response latencies in the arms and legs (25 to 50 ms). Latencies this rapid can be viewed as automatic and "hard-wired" and are probably the most rapidly responsive components to the perception of a stressor.

Another pathway that has been postulated is that of a stress-induced muscular patterning often called splinting, or bracing. The most thorough description of this theoretical perspective was given by Whatmore and Kohli (1974) who coined the term "disponesis" for maladaptive muscular bracing in functional disorders. In light of the current knowledge of muscle described in Part II, the automatic nature of the muscle patterns must be reexamined. However, even if the cortex can override specific muscular patterning, the splinting, or bracing, response may still be of importance.[6]

Part II: Consequences of Prolonged Activation of the Stress Response

Systems

In this section, I focus on the consequences of prolonged activation in a few of the described systems. This topic has been extensively explored, but often with insufficient data to confirm strong conclusions. The emphasis here is on the basis for models of psychophysiological disorders, that is, disorders in which there is evidence for a pathway starting with psychological or emotional constructs interacting with physiological mediators and finally influencing physical symptoms. A related pathway may exist for psychological symptoms such as panic, anxiety, or depression. These are considered when some peripheral mechanism is thought to be involved.

Disorders Related to Sympathetic Pathways

As noted, the sympathetic pathways have become the focus of attention for most psychophysiologic disorders. It is only recently, however, that concrete evidence for physiological mediators between symptoms and

---

[6] Bracing from stress or disponesis may underlie the pain experienced by voice patients with muscle tension disorders, as well as upper body muscular pain reported by performers with anticipatory anxiety related to communication apprehension. (B. H.)

psychological factors has been found. Two groups of disorders are worth emphasis: muscle pain disorders and irritable bowel syndrome (IBS).

Muscle pain has been presumed to be related to stress in the environment, but the presumed mechanisms were either unknown or systematically eliminated. Factors such as fatigue, microtrauma, spasm, or posture have been thought to be the pain mediators. Evidence for these pathways has been absent or at least not convincingly confirmed. Starting with the pioneering work of Janet Travell and David Simons (1983), it has been increasingly recognized that the "trigger point" represents a good candidate for muscle pain mechanisms. Trigger points (TPs) are small nodules imbedded in the muscle body that are tender to touch and refer pain to a characteristic area, sometimes distant from the TP, itself. As mentioned earlier, I have been able to show electromyographically that the trigger points are activated (or shut down) by alpha sympathetic pathways. This then paves the way for a true psychophysiological model of chronic muscle pain. Various emotional, or stressful, stimuli drive the activity in the TP for a long enough time to create the conditions for pain. It is hypothesized that this occurs in the muscle spindle, the sensory component of the muscle, but this remains speculative (See Simons, 1996). The role of bracing or splinting (disponesis) in this model is still unclear. Muscle response in the form of extrafusal contraction in the face of a stressor has been commonly observed (e.g, Whatmore & Kohli, 1974). In the experimental environment used in my needle TP studies, this response is not consistently seen. Perhaps the presence of a needle in the muscle overrides the usual motor reactions.

Our current efforts involve tracing the pathway to determine the psychological or perceptual stimuli most often involved, to flesh out the exact physiological pathways. It is suspected that situations involving interpersonal conflict, fear of negative self-evaluation, and lack of assertiveness play an important role. At this juncture, the work points the way to understanding muscle pain, at least partly as a psychophysiological disorder. This view, of course, has treatment (Gevirtz, Hubbard, & Harpin, 1997), as well as research implications.[7]

Another disorder that appears to be a sympathetically mediated psychophysiological disorder is irritable bowel syndrome (IBS). This disorder accounts for almost 50% of all gastroenterology referrals. Because there is typically no evidence of medical pathology, it is often thought by physicians to be a psychological disorder. However, studies by Drossman's group (Drossman et al., 1990) and others have found no real sign of psychopathology in most IBS sufferers. They do note that there is a subgroup of "medical seekers" who do appear to have significant psychosocial problems with frequent histories of abuse. A research group at

---

[7] Including implications for patients with "functional" voice disorders (B. H.)

UCLA led by Emeran Mayer (Bernstein et al., 1996; Lembo et al.,1994) have pioneered a psychophysiological model that emphasizes brain-gut interactions. Using balloon distension techniques in the colon, they have been able to show that IBS patients have hypersensitivity mediated by splanchnic afferents.

Blanchard & Malamoud (1996) have recently reviewed data that show that treatment of chronic worry or rumination in IBS patients is quite effective in reducing symptoms. These studies suggest a mediator path that would begin to explain IBS as another psychophysiological disorder. Processes associated with ruminative worry seem to disrupt the normal brain-gut regulation and, in addition, potentiate pain amplification through sympathetic splanchnic afferents [in the viscera]. Interventions that help to reregulate these systems seem to alleviate symptoms. For example, more than 60 years ago Jacobson (1938) reported using "progressive relaxation," a well-known means of reducing sympathetic activity, to successfully treat IBS.

The SNS is undoubtedly involved in many other disorders, as well. Research identifying mediators is just beginning, however. Disorders that are good candidates are: migraine headache, dermatological conditions, flare-ups of diseases such as inflammatory bowel disease and lupus, aspects of cardiovascular disease, panic disorder, and similar conditions.

Treatment Implications

The specificity of sympathetic pathways may imply that distinctive psychosocial stimuli may be involved for each organ system. This would lead to treatment protocols that target the specific psychophysiologic pathway. The two examples provided have evolved as our knowledge of the disorders has increased. For muscle pain, treatment relies on the pathway reaching back from the "spindle spasm" to the sympathetic innervation to psychological/emotional factors such as difficulty with assertion, avoidance of conflict, or fear of criticism. For IBS, it has been noted that autonomic pathways to the gut are interrupted by chronic stressors, such as worry or rumination.

As other distinct pathways emerge, treatment protocols will become more specific and, thus, more effective. This conceptualization may be distinguished from mass action arousal syndromes.

Disorders Related to Parasympathetic Nervous System Dysregulation

Although the PNS is probably involved in many aspects of health and disease, it is of primary interest in two major areas: life-sustaining cardiopulmonary regulation and bronchial asthma.

Several authors have documented the role of the vagal systems in sudden respiratory failure (Fox & Porges, 1985), recovery of acute myocardial infarction (Bigger et al., 1988), and hypertension (Malliani, Pagani, Lombardi, & Cerutti, 1991). In this regard, Porge's idea of the reciprocal relationship between the smart and vegetative vagus is salient. The idea that more subtle influences may be at work in other disorders underlies the role of the PNS in bronchial asthma.

Asthma is characterized by excessive bronchial airway reactivity, usually in response to an allergen or external irritant. A great deal is now known about the histamine and mast cell mechanisms at the end point of the reaction. Much less is known about the autonomic systems involved. It is known that the SNS plays only a minor role in actual airway regulation and that the bronchospastic reaction is mediated by the PNS. It has been recognized that there is a subset of asthmatics in whom an attack can be triggered by emotional or stressful situations. It was assumed that the PNS plays a role, but the mechanism had been unclear (Lehrer, Eisenberg, & Hochron, 1993). Most research is pointing toward subtle dysregulation of the SNS/PNS balance, especially following prolonged stress. Heeren and associates (Heeren, Gevirtz, & Seltzer, 1997) have found that asthmatics with emotionally triggered attacks show a more pronounced RSA response after a stressor than do asthmatics with nonemotionally triggered attacks. Similarly, Sturani, Sturani, & Tosi (1985) found that intrinsic asthma patients (those without common allergies), showed an exaggerated bradycardia (heart rate decrease) response to a cold stimulus on the face (diving reflex), compared to nonasthma patients. This would seem to indicate a dominance in the vegetative vagus, possibly through smart vagal withdrawal. In any case, this research points the way toward including autonomic responses to stress in our understanding of asthma.[8]

Treatment Implications

Lehrer (1997) has recently written an essay describing the possible advantages of using nonlinear models (chaos analysis) in assessing ANS homeostasis or lack thereof. It may be that our newfound interest in PNS will lead to more productive treatment models for disorders such as panic, asthma, hypertension, motion sickness, and so on than was possible with more linear models.

Lehrer's emphasis on "oscillators" may be generlizable to disorders, such as chronic fatigue or fibromyalgia, where evidence exists for stress having a long-term disruptive effect on chronobiological oscillations.

---

[8] This research may also relate to the etiology of certain types of paradoxical vocal cord dysfunction (PVCD). (B. H.)

Treatments in this instance would be targeted to restoring the proper mix of rhythms, be they circadian, utradian,[9] or very-low-frequency cardiovascular oscillations. As an example, Lehrer et al. (1997) describe a form of RSA biofeedback long used in Russia for asthma treatment. The underlying rationale is daily recalibration of low-frequency cardiac cycles through biofeedback exercises. In this pilot study, such training produced dramatic lung function improvements as compared to a normal relaxation type of treatment. Similarly, Herbs and Gevirtz (1994) found that RSA biofeedback training was as effective as finger temperature training in reducing blood pressure in hypertensives. In this model, the training is conceptualized not as only enhancing vagal tone, but as a method of restoring disordered dynamic homeostatic systems.

Respiratory Factors as Mediators of Psychophysiological and Anxiety Disorders

Respiratory responses to stress are emerging as good candidates for mediators of symptoms in a variety of stress-related and anxiety disorders. The mechanisms of subtle hyperventilation and the systemic sequelae that affect a wide variety of organ systems appear to explain at least some of the variance in a number of disorders such as functional cardiac disorder, panic, some phobias, and general somatization disorders.

Functional cardiac disorder is a common classification used by cardiologists and internists to describe patients with symptoms such as chest pain, dyspnea, dizziness, and so on, but without measurable medical pathology. We (DeGuire, Gevirtz, Hawkinson, & Dixon, 1996; DeGuire, Gevirtz, Kawahara, & Maguire, 1992) have shown that these patients, often with low normal end tidal carbon dioxide ($ETCO_2$) and rapid respiration rate, decrease their symptoms dramatically when trained in slow diaphragmatic breathing. The rate of symptom reduction is highly and significantly correlated with normalization of breathing parameters ($r = .59$), indicating the probable role of respiration as a mediator of chest symptoms.

Breathing anomalies may help explain some aspects of anxiety disorders such as panic disorder. The role of hyperventilation in panic disorder has been hotly debated (cf. Papp, Klein, & Gorman,1993). Some of the contradictory findings could be explained by the existence of subgroups among these patients. Ronald Ley (1992) has proposed three such subgroups, ranging from those with heavy respiratory and physiological involvement to those with mostly cognitive distortion. Of interest here is the proposed existence of a respiratory subgroup with frequent "out of the blue" attacks.

[9] high-frequency and pulsatile

We (Moynihan & Gevirtz, 1996) have found that the out of the blue, or spontaneous, subtype patients had lower $ETCO_2$, indicating a possible mechanism through which frequent overbreathing could produce symptoms.

Fried (1993) described many other disorders with possible respiratory mediation.

Treatment Implications

Treatment implications connected with respiratory psychophysiology have been discussed for many years. Robert Fried (1993) discussed the far-ranging physical and psychological consequences of hyperventilation (both acute and chronic) in great detail. The International Society for the Advancement of Respiratory Psychophysiology (ISARP) has focused on respiratory psychophysiological topics for more than 10 years. Timmons and Ley (1994) also have many chapters devoted to the clinical applications of respiratory phenomena.

A consensus of most clinicians in this area is that almost all psychophysiological and some anxiety disorder treatment protocols should start with breathing retraining. Since this has been the basis of virtually every Eastern meditative art for thousands of years, this seems to be a safe recommendation.

Disorders Related to Endocrine Dysregulation

It has long been assumed that prolonged secretion of glucocorticoids has deleterious health consequences. This was the primary implication of the concept of the "exhaustion" stage of Selye's GAS (1974). Ulcers were noted as the prototypical disease that results from this prolonged "exhaustion" of the endocrine system. Since this early conceptualization, many other diseases and syndromes have been hypothesized to be the result of excessive glucocorticoid production in response to environmental demands. For example, corticosteroids have been postulated to be involved in the development of atherosclerosis, elevated serum lipids, and increased proportion of dead or injured endothelial cells (Henry, 1983). This pathway is proposed over and above a sympathoadrenal medullary involvement in lipid mobilization (Havel & Goldstein, 1959). More recent efforts have focused on hostility as the "active ingredient in cardiovascular disease, with glucocorticoids playing an important, but not exclusive, role (Suarez & Williams, 1992).

It has long been recognized that stress, especially if chronic and uncontrollable, can affect immune function. From these early observations, the field of psychoimmunology has emerged. Humoral and cellular immune responses have been extensively studied in laboratory and naturalistic settings. Findings have generally been interpreted to indicate that a lowered immune function will occur after stress. Although most people under stress do not become ill, when other vulnerabilities and risk factors exist, the stress/hormonal/immune connection becomes important. This topic is beyond the scope of the present chapter but has been covered in a book entitled *Human Stress and Immunity*, edited by Ronald Glaser and Janice Keicolt-Glaser (1994).

Chapter Summary

This chapter described the fundamental physiological responses to stress. I have emphasized the autonomic, endocrine, and immune systems in an effort to provide an understanding of the pathways through which especially prolonged stress might affect the body. Understanding these pathways may help us to understand psychophysiological disorders. This is a significant task from a public health point of view, because the disorders described account for a large proportion of health care resource utilization. With the dwindling resources available, it is clear that improving the understanding of the impact of stress on the body will produce large dividends both from a humane and financial point of view.

References

Barker, D. & Banks, R. (1986). The muscle spindle. In A. Engel & B. Banker (Eds.), *Myology* (pp. 309–341). New York: McGraw-Hill.

Bernstein, C., Niazi, N., Robert, M., Mertz, H., Kodner, A., Munakata, J., Naliboff, B., & Mayer, E. (1996). Rectal afferent function in patients with inflammatory and functional intestinal disorders. *Pain, 66,* 151–161.

Bernston, G., Cacioppo, J., & Quigley, K. (1993). Respiratory sinus arrhythmia: Autonomic origins, physiological mechanisms, and psychophysiological implications. *Psychophysiology, 30,* 183–196.

Bickford, R., Jacboson, J., & Cody, D. (1964). Nature of average evoked potentials to sound and other stimuli in men. *Annals of the New York Academy of Sciences, 112,* 204–210.

Bigger, J., Kleiger, R., Fleiss, J., Rolnitzky, L., Steinman, R., & Miller, J. (1988). Components of heart rate variability measure during healing of acute myocardial infarction. *American Journal of Cardiology, 61,* 208–215.

Blanchard, E. & Malamoud, H. (1996). Psychological treatment of irritable bowel syndrome. *Professional Psychology, 27,* 241–244.

Cohen, S. (1992). Stress, social support & disorder. In H. O. F. Veiel & U. Baumann (Eds.), *The meaning and measurement of social support* (pp. 109–124). New York: Hemisphere Publishing Corp.

Cummins, S., & Gevirtz, R. N. (1992). The relationship between daily stress and urinary cortisol in a normal population: An emphasis on individual differences. *Behavioral Medicine, 19,* 129–134.

Davis, W. (1983) *The degree of perceptual salience and perceptual difficulty on covert oral responses.* Unpublished doctoral dissertation, University of Louisville, KY.

DeGuire, S., Gevirtz, R., Hawkinson, D., & Dixon, K. (1996). Breathing retraining: A three-year follow-up study of treatment for hyperventilation syndrome and associated functional cardiac symptoms. *Biofeedback and Self-Regulation, 21,* 191–198.

DeGuire, S., Gevirtz, R. N., Kawahara, Y., & Maguire, W. (1992) Hyperventilation syndrome and the assessment of treatment for functional cardiac symptoms. *American Journal of Cardiology, 70,* 673–677.

Drossman, D., Thompson, G., Talley, N., Funch-Jensen, P., Jansens, J., & Whitehead, W. (1990). Identification of subgroups of functional gastrointestinal disorders. *Gastroenterology International, 3,* 159–172.

Eckberg, D. & Sleight, P. (1992). *Human baroreflexes in health and disease.* Oxford: Clarendon Press.

Fox, N. & Porges, S. (1985). The relation between neonatal heart period patterns and developmental outcome. *Child Development, 56,* 28–37.

File, S. E., Vellucci, S. V., & Wendlandt, S. (1979) Corticosterone—An anxiogenic or anxiolytic agent? *Journal of Pharmacy and Pharmacology, 31,* 300–305.

Freedman, R. R. (1991). Physiological mechanisms of temperature biofeedback. *Biofeedback and Self-Regulation, 16,* 95–115.

Freedman, R. R., Sabharwal, S. C., Ianni, P., Nagaraj, D., Wenig, P., & Mayes, M. D. (1988). Nonneural beta-adrenergic vasodilating mechanism in temperature biofeedback. *Psychosomatic Medicine, 50,* 394–401.

Fried, R. (1993). *The psychology and physiology of breathing.* New York: Plenum.

Fukado, S., Lane, J., Anderson, N., Kuhn, C., Schanberg, S., McCown, N., Muranaka, M., Suzuki, J., & Williams, R. (1989). Vagal antagonism of cardiovascular and electrophysiologic responses to isoproterenol infusion is weaker in Type A than Type B men. Paper presented at the annual meeting of the American Psychosomatic Society, San Francisco.

Gevirtz, R., Hubbard, D., & Harpin, R. E. (1996). Psychophysiologic treatment of chronic lower back pain. *Professional Psychology: Research and Practice, 27,* 561–566.

Glaser, R., & Kiecolt-Glaser, J. (Eds.). (1994). *Human stress and immunity.* San Diego: Academic Press.

Gold, P., Goodwin, F., & Chrousos, G. (1988). Clinical and biochemical manifestations of depression. Part 1. *New England Journal of Medicine, 319,* 348–353.

Guyton, A. (1976). *Structure and function of the nervous system.* Philadelphia: W. B. Saunders Co.

Guyton, A., & Hall, J. (1995). *Textbook of medical physiology* (9th ed.). Philadelphia: W. B. Saunders Co.

Han, J. N., Stegan, K., Simkens, K., Canberghs, M., Schepers, R., Van den Bergh, D., Clement, J., & Van de Woestijine, K. (1997). Unsteadiness of breathing in patients with hyperventilation syndrome and anxiety disorders. *European Respiratory Journal, 10,* 167–176.

Havel, R. & Goldstein, A. (1959). The role of the sympathetic nervous system in the metabolism of free fatty acids. *Journal of Lipid Research, 1,* 102–108.

Heeren, M., Gevirtz, R., & Seltzer, J. (1996, March). *Psychophysiological response patterns in emotionally triggered asthma.* Poster session presented at the 28th annual meeting of the Association for Applied Psychophysiology and Biofeedback, San Diego.

Henry, J. (1983). Coronary heart disease and arousal of the adrenal cortical axis. In T. M. Dembrowski & T. Schmidt (Eds.), *Bio-behavioral basis of coronary heart disease.* Basel, Switzerland: Karger.

Herbs, D., Gevirtz, R., & Jacobs, D. (1994). The effect of heart rate pattern biofeedback for the treatment of essential hypertension. Paper presented at the 25th annual meeting of the Association for Applied Psychophysiology and Biofeedback, Atlanta.

Hubbard, D. & Berkoff, G. (1993). Myofascial trigger points show spontaneous needle EMG activity. *Spine, 18,* 1803–1807.

Jacobson, E. (1938). *Progressive relaxation* (rev. ed.). Chicago: University of Chicago Press.

Jänig, W. & McLachlan, E. (1992). Specialized functional pathways are building blocks of the autonomic nervous system. *Journal of the Autonomic Nervous System, 41,* 3–14.

Lazarus, R., & Folkman, S. (1984). *Stress, appraisal, and coping.* New York: Springer.

Lehrer, P. (1997). Chaos, catastrophe, oscillation, and self-regulation [book review and essay]. *Applied Psychophysiology and Biofeedback, 22,* 215–223.

Lehrer, P., Carr, R., Smetankin, E., Vaschillo, E., Peper, E., Porges, S., Eckberg, R., Hamer, R., & Hochron, S. (1997). Respiratory sinus arrhythmia versus neck/trapezious EMG and incentive inspirometry biofeedback for asthma: a pilot study. *Applied Psychophysiology and Biofeedback, 22,* 95–109.

Lehrer, P., Eisenberg, S., & Hochron, S. (1993). Asthma and emotion: A review. *Journal of Asthma, 30,* 5–21.

Lembo, T., Munakata, J., Mentz, H., Niazi, N., Kodner, A., Nikas, V., & Mayer, E. (1994). Evidence for the hypersensitivity of lumbar splanchnic afferents in irritable bowel syndrome. *Gastroenterology, 107,* 1686–1696.

Ley, R. (1992). The many faces of pain: Psychological and physiological differences among three types of panic attacks. *Behavior Research and Therapy, 30,* 347–357.

Malliani, A., Pagani, M., Lombardi, F., & Cerutti, S. (1991). Clinical and experimental evaluation of sympatho-vagal interaction: Power spectral analysis of heart rate and arterial pressure variabilities. In I. H. Zucker & J. P. Gilmore (Eds.), *The reflex control of circulation* (pp. 937–964). Boca Raton, FL: CRC Press.

Mayer, E. & Gebhart, G. (1994). Basic and clinical aspects of visceral hyperalgesia. *Gastroenterology, 107,* 271–293.

Mayer, E. & Rayboud, H. (1990). Role of visceral hyperalgesia. *Gastroenterology, 99,* 1688–1704.

McEwen, B. & Mendelson, S. (1993). Effects of stress on the neurochemistry and morphology of the brain: Counterregulation versus damage. In L. Goldberger & S. Breznitz (Eds.), *Handbook of stress* (2nd ed) (pp. 101–126). New York: The Free Press.

McGuigan, F. J. (1978). *Cognitive psychophysiology: Principles of covert behavior.* Englewood Cliffs, NJ: Prentice Hall.

McNulty, W., Gevirtz, R., Hubbard, D., & Berkoff, G. (1994). Needle electromyographic evaluation of trigger point response to a psychological stressor. *Psychophysiology, 31,* 313–316.

Moynihan, J. & Gevirtz, R. (1996). Towards identifying subtypes of panic using respiratory and psychophysiologic factors: A preliminary investigation (abstract). *Biological Psychology, 43,* 253.

Munck, A., Guyre, P., & Holbrook, N. (1984). Physiological function of glucocorticoids in stress and their relation to pharmacological actions. *Endocrinology Review, 5,* 25–44.

Muranaka, M., Monou, H., Suzuki, J., Lane, J. D., Anderson, N. B., Kuhn, C. M., Schanberg, S. M., McCown, N., & Williams, R. B., Jr. (1988). Physiological responses to catecholamine infusions in type A and type B men. *Health Psychology, 7* (suppl.), 145–163.

Papp, L., Klein, D., & Gorman, J. (1993). Carbon dioxide hypersensitivity, hyperventilation, and panic disorder. *American Journal of Psychiatry, 150,* 1149–1157.

Passatore, M., Filippi, M., & Grassi, C. (1985). Cervical sympathetic nerve stimulation can induce an intrafusal muscle fibre contraction in the rabbit. In I. Body & M. Gadden (Eds.), *The muscle spindle* (pp. 221–226). London: Macmillan.

Porges, S. (1995). Orienting in a defensive world: Mammalian modifications of our evolutionary heritage. A polyvagal theory. *Psychophysiology, 32*, 301–318.

Saffran, M. & Dokas, L. (1983). Sites of nonspecificity in the response of the adrenocortical system to stress. In H. Selye (Ed.), *Selye's guide to stress research* (Vol. 3). New York: Scientific and Academic Editions.

Schore, A. (1994). *Affect regulation and the origin of the self.* Hillsdale, NJ: Lawrence Erlbaum.

Selye, H. (1936). Non-specificity of the pituitary-adrenocortical system to stress. *Nature, 138*, 32.

Selye, H. (1956). *The stress of life.* New York: McGraw-Hill.

Selye, H. (1973). The evolution of the stress concept. *American Scientist, 61*, 692–699.

Selye, H. (1974). *Stress without distress.* Philadelphia: J. P. Lippincott.

Simons, D. (1996). Clinical and etiological update of myofascial pain from trigger points. *Journal of Musculoskeletal Pain, 4*, 93–121.

Sturani, C., Sturani, A., & Tosi, I. (1985). Parasympathetic activity assessed by diving reflex and by airway response to methacholine in bronchial asthma and rhinitis. *Respiration, 48*, 321–328.

Suarez, E. & Williams, R. (1992). Interactive models of reactivity: The relationship between hostility and potentially pathogenic physiological responses to social stressors. In N. Schneiderman, P. McCabe, & A. Baum (Eds.), *Perspectives in behavioral medicine: Stress and disease processes* (pp. 175–195). Hillsdale, NJ: Lawrence Erlbaum Associates.

Timmons, B. & Ley, R. (Eds.). (1994). *Behavioral and psychological approaches to breathing disorders.* Plenum Press: New York.

Travell, J. & Simons, D. (1983–1992). *Myofascial pain and dysfunction: The trigger point manual* (vols. 1–2). Baltimore: Williams & Wilkins.

Whatmore, G. & Kohli, D. (1974). *The physiopathology and treatment of functional disorders.* New York: Grune & Statton.

Ursin, H., Baade, E., & Levine, S. (1978). *Psychobiology of stress: A study of coping man.* New York: Academic Press.

CHAPTER

5

Management Perspectives

COMMUNICATION APPREHENSION REDUCTION PROGRAMS

The need for professional help to alleviate communication apprehension/performance anxiety is finally being recognized. In the past, a few research centers such as Hahneman Medical School, the New York Psychiatric Institute, Stanford University, and Southern Indiana University, as well as some private psychologists, have offered services for the social phobics who managed to find treatment facilities. Today, other universities and some professional schools recognize the seriousness of the problem and are offering seminars to help performing artists overcome their performance fears. This includes Julliard School of Performing Arts, Curtis School of Music, Yale, Oberlin College, Northwestern University, and the New World Symphony in Miami Beach seminars. This is heartening for the aspiring and performing artists who have not conquered their fear of performance. However, there are millions of ordinary, even extraordinary, people also suffering from the related problem of communication apprehension for whom services are not readily available. This population is far greater than all the professional performers and patients with disorders combined. It includes people in business and the professions, as well as athletes and students. Whatever the challenge—artistic, business, or social—the fear of fear and of humiliation, embarrassment, and helplessness is at the core of performance anxiety.

This chapter presents one program for communication apprehension/performance anxiety that is primarily for business and professional people called Speaking Without Fear and conducted at a large, urban university. However, the program can be easily adapted to other populations in education, corporations, and agencies, as well as the performing arts for communication apprehension is an equal-opportunity fear reaction. Its root causes and debilitating effects are shared equally by stage stars, athletes, office workers, professionals, high-powered executives, and students. The mind-body connection is at the heart of it all. Consequently, management strategies are similar for all types of performance anxiety.

The Speaking Without Fear program incorporates and reflects most of the information on the origins of communication apprehension discussed in this book. It also combines the intervention strategies found to be effective with anxiety disorders (See Chapter 3) with other approaches found valuable by the author (B. H.) in defusing the mythology and inordinate reactions of people suffering from communication apprehension.

Comments by students prior to enrolling in the Speaking Without Fear course reflect the feelings of most participants in the program:

> I have been living with the fear of public speaking for as long as I can remember. All through adolescence I dreaded school assignments that required oral presentations. I hated being watched by others for I was certain I would do or say something to make a complete fool of myself. Such feeling of dread was often accompanied by shaking hands, quivering voice, inability to make eye contact, etc. As such experiences continued, and with each opportunity to experience what I considered failure, I soon compounded my fear of public speaking with rejection and absolute disappointment in myself. The physical nervous behavior was followed by an inner voice that nagged me for being nervous.
>
> I am now an adult, and my vain attempts to control my fear on my own have proven fruitless. In the fall I noticed a class being offered that dealt with the fear of public speaking. I certainly feel it is time for me to ask for help.
>
> **Allison**

> At work I am plagued by feelings of anxiety whenever I am asked to speak in front of a group or on a conference call with more than four people. I find that I avoid these situations as much as possible and since I've always been a good artist, I rely on creating images that "speak" for me, while others present ideas verbally. Since I'm in the design field, this reliance on images works fine but I also realize that I

can never grow to the next level career-wise and personally if I cannot present my own ideas verbally.

Norman

I am taking the time to write this e-mail because I believe my situation is unique. I stutter. I am involved in speech therapy and am making wonderful progress, but something left over from years of dysfluency is an irrational fear involved with speaking in front of others. I want it gone!! I am hoping that you can offer me some advice on a course which fits my needs.

Nicholas

COURSE OVERVIEW

Group or Individual Format?

Although the problem of communication apprehension can be managed individually, a small group is the most effective treatment format for several reasons. First, the presence of other group members dispels the mistaken notion that people with communication apprehension are unique, thereby facilitating self-disclosure, an important first step in diffusing the problem.

Second, a group provides the stressful environment necessary for the desensitization of speakers' fears, as well as an opportunity to receive objective feedback that refutes erroneous beliefs, perceptions, and thoughts.

Third, the participants provide support and reassurance to each other that is often more convincing than words from even the most effective facilitator.

Fourth, the heterogeneity of a group consisting of participants of varying ethnic backgrounds, genders, ages, and vocations makes the experience interesting. It enables participants to appreciate the universality of communication apprehension that transcends academic, cultural, or class distinctions. It also elicits humor, a great stress reducer, as people demystify their respective paper tigers.

Fifth, participants learn from observing others that responding to challenge (usually considered stress) with arousal is natural and not all bad, and to consider the eustress, distress, and optimal stress phenomena as illustrated in Figure 5-1, Types of Stress (Everly & Rosenfeld, 1981). Eustress is a positive form of stress that is motivating. Distress is

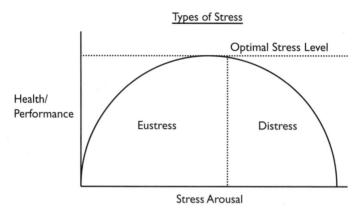

FIGURE 5-1. From *The Nature and Treatment of the Stress Response: A Practical Guide for Clinicians* (p. 7), by G. S. Everly, Jr., and R. Rosenfeld, 1981, New York: Plenum Press. Copyright 1981 by Plenum Press. Reprinted with permission.

the point at which positive stress turns negative from overload or lack of stress or challenge. The optimal stress point for an individual level is where stress is maximally productive.

Finally, the group format elicits discussions of feelings, attitudes, and beliefs that often evoke repressed memories that are at the core of a participant's communication apprehension. It also enables acknowledgement and affirmation of everyone's personal growth over time. In short, it helps set and keep records straight.

Course Details

Speaking Without Fear is a noncredit course at the School of Continuing and Professional Studies at New York University that is offered three times a year with a maximum of 16 students. The 3-hour class meets once weekly in the evening for eight consecutive weeks. A variety of other formats also have been offered, including 6- and 10-week sessions, with adjustments made in the length of individual sessions. Follow-up booster sessions also have been given and found effective in reinforcing the positive attitudes and skills gained during the course. The booster sessions, too, have varied formats, including intensive weekend classes (3 hours, Saturday and Sunday) for two consecutive weeks, four weekly meetings of 2 hours duration, and/or individual therapy sessions.

Participants in the group are generally educated and upwardly mobile. They include people in varied careers at all levels, including business, banking, law, medicine, psychology, computer technology, the sciences, the visual and performing arts, journalism, and graduate education. Ages range from the mid-20s to the mid-70s, with an equal number of men and women, from all parts of the world. All have serious communication blocks professionally, often personally as well, and generally have not addressed their communication apprehension in any academic forum nor disclosed their fears to anyone. Rather, they have expended psychic energy hiding, avoiding, or suffering at great personal cost. Enrollment in the course is a major step for them, perhaps their most difficult. However, once they see and meet others in the same boat, they feel immediate relief and hope.

Course Purpose

The overall purpose of the course is fourfold: (1) to clarify the biological and psychological etiology of communication apprehension; (2) to facilitate a variety of coping strategies including cognitive, behavioral, physiological, and affective; (3) to provide students with experience by having them gradually confront the feared situations they have painfully endured or scrupulously avoided; and (4) to develop communication skills related to a variety of speaking tasks in different contexts. Hence, the overall goal of the course is to understand the mind-body connection and to facilitate strategies and experiences that reduce or overcome speaking fears.

Cognitive targets include (1) demystifying communication apprehension through an explanation of the mind-body connection, (2) restructuring cognitions—and reformulating negativity into positive thoughts, (3) defusing semantic triggers and cultural hooks that bind and blind people, (4) using positive verbal/mental cues, and (5) tracking thoughts, feelings, and progress.

Physiological targets consist of autogenic training, that is, self-regulation techniques, including diaphragmatic breathing, heart rate control, and neuromuscular relaxation exercises with the aid of simple biofeedback instrumentation. They also include centering techniques, which incorporate awareness of attention and correct breathing patterns combined with positive cues and visual imagery. Information on the relationship of nutrition and stress is also presented.

Affective targets include releasing feelings such as fears and feelings of success, developing insights, gaining support and reassurance, acquiring realistic self-perceptions, and identification or transference with the facilitator/clinician, an integral aspect of every clinical relationship.

Experiential targets include reducing escapism, desensitization by gradually doing what is feared, and speaking immersion.

Communication skill targets include learning the anatomy of presentations and effective rehearsal and delivery techniques, with individual assessment and training as needed. When necessary, other targets include referrals for psychotherapy, voice or speech therapy, or medical examination.

Students are expected to attend all sessions, because class assignments are hierarchically arranged to reduce stress. That is, speaking tasks are gradually increased in difficulty and presented in varied communicative contexts and physical settings. Participants must also complete homework assignments, which include questionnaires and a bibliotherapy aimed at developing insight into the nature of individual fears. Students are encouraged to personalize the program, for only they know which management strategies are most effective in helping them to feel centered, focused, and in control. They are also expected to practice self-regulation techniques at home, gradually increase their participation in feared situations outside of class, and maintain records of their practice and reactions to class assignments in a journal. Hence, participants assume responsibility for their progress.

Participants provide their own tapes for videotaping of formal oral presentations in class and view them at home. No grades are assigned in the course, except when requested by students whose companies reimburse employees for outside training. This practice relieves students from the stress of evaluations, a major part of communication anxiety in the first place, and frees the instructor from arbitrary judgments of performances.

Class Communication Climate

Initially, tension is very high, because class members do not know what to expect in the first group meeting. Therefore, it is important to establish an ambiance conducive to trust and open communication. A U-shaped arrangement of chairs helps provide this positive climate because it enables eye contact with all participants and a sense of equality with everyone, including the facilitator. It also encourages participation, because there is no place for anyone to hide. Later in the class the stress level can be increased by placing the chairs in a more traditional or formal classroom or auditorium arrangement.

However, the most important element in establishing a positive communication climate for any performance anxiety program is the group leader. It is preferable to consider group leaders as facilitators, because their most important role is to facilitate the growth of individuals struggling with a host of negative thoughts and distressing physiological symptoms that impede natural abilities. Hence, facilitators, like Zen masters, should be role models who set the tone in a supportive and nonjudgmental way. If the facilitator has actually overcome their own inordinate fears of performance, whatever its nature, his or her credibility will be enormously enhanced, for the mind-body issues of communication apprehension are similar in all endeavors: sports, speaking, professional performances, and vocalizing. However, being a performer without having suffered the problem or only having conquered the fear may not be enough. At best, it requires both knowledge and personal experience. Nevertheless, some individuals with more sensitivity and intuition than information or personal history can be effective facilitators.

Whatever their background, facilitators must be teachers who explain the origins of communication apprehension and demystify the voodoo surrounding the problem. They must also be observers of distorted thinking, diplomats in reformulating negative thoughts, trainers who explain and demonstrate coping strategies to reduce hyperarousal, and coaches who effectively shape skills related to specific types of performances. Above all, facilitators must be patient, reassuring, realistic, and scientific: a kind of detective who is willing to help others sort out pieces of a fearful puzzle. It also takes knowledge and sensitivity to recognize which problems they can help resolve, skill to help people help themselves, and realism to recognize those in need of referrals to other professionals. Communication apprehension is a serious problem that warrants a high level of professionalism. Facilitating groups of people suffering from this problem is a significant and gratifying professional responsibility.

Openness is probably the best way for a facilitator to establish immediate credibility and a positive communication climate in the group. I have often likened teaching the classes in Speaking Without Fear to climbing Everest. In the dim past, I struggled with every trick of the trade—panicking, avoiding, and rationalizing when it came to making presentations in public—although throughout my school life and afterward, I was able to act in plays where I assumed roles. This confession has proven helpful to students (and clients) who invariably report how reassuring that message is, because they believe that they are alone in their fears, and cannot imagine that their professor or clinician ever had a problem or that anyone could conquer fears that seemed so insurmountable. One student was so impressed with my sporting analogy about climbing Mt Everest that he took it literally and bragged to his friends about his "mountain climber" instructor!

Obviously, one need not be an expert mountain climber or Olympic champion to use sports examples to set the tone of a group. I have also revealed my frustrations as a former skier who reached a plateau at the intermediate level because of fears that caused me to tense up on more advanced trails. It wasn't until I found myself on a wind-swept mountaintop on a bitter cold day, desperate to get off quickly, that I skied down an expert trail—the most direct route to the warm and inviting clubhouse. For the first time in my skiing career I was truly focused and relied on my instinctive knowledge of the sport and balance rather than being worried about falling. My objective was crystal clear. I did not even try! It just flowed. A great feeling!

A similar experience occurred when I was playing tennis. I played fairly well, but fell apart when someone watched me. As soon as I became aware of being observed, my mind became cluttered with negative thoughts that interfered with my coordination! These true stories and others have been extremely effective in establishing trust, identification, and credibility with groups and individuals working to overcome their fear of performance and communication. Facilitators should encourage students to reflect on their own sports experiences as examples of the mind-body connection. Students should also be informed about professional athletes and performers who have learned to constructively control and channel their performance fears (See Chapter 1).

Class Agenda

The following is a typical agenda for the 8-week course, which includes maximum speaking opportunities in each session. Individual videotapings of student oral presentations are made in the later five sessions and viewed at home.

Class I

Class 1 begins with an icebreaker and introductions. Seated in a semicircle, students are immediately instructed to introduce themselves to their neighbors and to learn about them, especially their reasons for taking the class. The purpose of this interaction is for each participant to gain enough information about the other to introduce him or her to the group. This icebreaker is helpful in reducing the tension of the first speaking experience in the group because each person's focus is on someone else rather than themselves. After 10 minutes of interactions, volunteers, who can remain seated, introduce their neighbors to the group. The facilitator encourages both parties to elaborate more about their backgrounds.

Immediately after speaking, participants are given a questionnaire, a Simply Noticing exercise (Appendix 5-1) rate their level of fear as well as record his or her thoughts and feelings while speaking. Participants are also requested to draw their fear and to give it a name. A discussion about participants' reactions to their first speaking experiences in the group is then facilitated.

This first round of introductions and subsequent discussion are very fruitful, because people learn about each other's reactions, backgrounds, and stress symptoms, which are usually not obvious to anyone but themselves. Invariably, people remark that everyone other than themself seems okay and express surprise that so many articulate and accomplished people struggle with a problem they thought was unique to them. They also recognize a commonality of ideas and attitudes.

The commonality among participants is the basis of further discussion. For example, in a recent class, five students admitted that they withheld telling anyone about enrolling in the course because they feared being considered weak or embarrassed. One corporate executive opted to pay for the course himself rather than request reimbursement from his training department, which would have paid for it. Another student whispered the name of the course in the phone to her supervisor rather than say it aloud, for fear others would overhear, while another simply lied to her boss about the name of the course. Paradoxically, the extreme measures that people took to cover up resulted in great relief, because everyone quickly recognized the absurdity and humor in the situation. This relief was further enhanced when they learned that communication apprehension, in particular speaking in public, is a top-rated fear and a normal reaction to threat, real or perceived. But most importantly, students speak up and out in a group, sometimes for the first time. They quickly realize that they are all in the same boat and begin pulling for each other. Inevitably some students are more courageous and test the waters even further, daring to stand up or come to the front of the room, if not in the first round of presentations, later. Others often follow.

Following the discussion, an orientation to the course and the agenda are explained, a student information form is distributed (Appendix 5-2), and several short personality tests are administered. The purpose of the tests is to determine the traits and thinking patterns of participants that may put them at risk for threat perception (See Wickramasekera discussion in Chapter 2) and to be able to evaluate and inform participants about aspects of their personality that put them at risk for somatizing their fears, resulting in communication apprehension. The tests administered include the short version of the Eysenck Personality Questionnaire (Eysenck & Eysenck, 1976), that assesses extroversion, emotional toughness, emotional lability, and lying (self-deception). Other tests include the Absorption Scale (Tellegen & Atkinson, 1974), which measures personality traits of suggestibility and sensitivity (related to hypnotizability), the Marlowe-Crown scale of self-deception or repression (Crown & Marlowe, 1960), and a Dysfunctional Cognitive Inventory, which measures a tendency to catastrophize (Zocco, 1984). Results of these tests, which are later explained to participants, are extremely helpful in clarifying each student's risk for threat perception and potential for coping under stress. Some of the personality traits are inherited (e.g., suggestability, introversion/extroversion) and others are learned (e.g., catastrophizing, self deception).

A Personal Report of Confidence as a Speaker (PRCS), which is a symptom inventory from Paul's 1966 *Insight vs. Desensitization in Psychotherapy* (as cited in Schneier & Welkowitz, 1996), is administered to get a baseline measure of the degree of nervousness in speaking in public. The class then breaks for 10 minutes, enabling students to interact and bond with each other, something that happens rather quickly.

Communication Model

The last half of the first class is a lecture on background information designed to dispel the mysticism about communication apprehension and the relationship of thinking to words. The lecture/discussion begins with a general model of communication that helps participants think in terms of communicating messages (verbal, vocal, and nonverbal) and expressing ideas rather than impressing anyone or giving speeches. The model applies to audiences of all sizes, one to one or a large group (Figure 5-2).

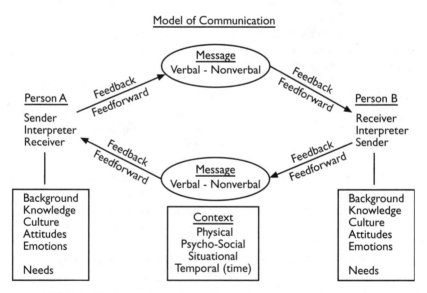

FIGURE 5-2. This model of communication illustrates the two-way nature of communication and the reciprocal influences of the continuous feedback loop of verbal and nonverbal messages in a communicative exchange. Each person in a communicative transaction is represented as a sender, interpreter, and receiver. Every message is subject to distortion or misunderstanding, as an individual with a background separate from the speaker interprets it based on knowledge, culture, and needs. Messages are also influenced by context.

Communication is explained as a two-way process in which the persons involved are simultaneously senders, interpreters, and receivers. The model suggests that communication consists of continuous, dynamic, reciprocal, and mutually influential verbal and nonverbal messages that are affected by the context in which the messages occur. The context includes the physical surroundings (room, place), psychosocial aspects (status, relationships), situational details (formality/informality), and temporal elements (length of time, time of day or evening). The reciprocal feedback of verbal and nonverbal messages by both sender and receiver regulates the communication process. The ability to give and receive feedback, as well as to be proactive, is a necessary skill for effective social interaction and communication. The more that is known about oneself, the listener, and the topic, the more effective communication is.

Students generally do not understand the relationship between thoughts, language, and speech nor do they know how speech is produced. Their misconceptions result in the belief that they must focus on words rather than on ideas when presenting informally in a group or that they can exercise no control over their tone, rate, or volume of speech. These mistaken notions often contribute to an individual's inordinate anxiety about speaking in public. For this reason a brief explanation of how language and speech are produced is presented.

According to the model of speech production shown in Figure 5-3 (Levelt, 1989; Peters, 1998), there are three main components involved in speaking. These include cognitive processes, language processes, and speech production. The cognitive processes involve the conceptualization of an idea for a message that is preverbal. This preverbal message is then transformed by language processes into syntactic and semantic forms (unspoken grammar and words). The next component is the speech production stage, which is motor planning and commands for muscle preparation and execution of the preverbal message that leads to the acoustic event known as speech.

Clarifying the process of speech production helps students with communication apprehension understand that they can rely on their ideas being transformed automatically into words. Understanding this concept generally relieves students from pre-selecting or fixating on specific words, something which actually impedes the flow of ideas. Focusing on ideas rather than words facilitates spontaneous communication and helps students express themselves with confidence.

The concept of social phobia (See Chapter 3) is then introduced and the characteristics and demographics of the problem are discussed. This information is usually received with considerable relief, especially when it is learned that there is a diagnosis for their problem, which is easily treated if understood. A discussion of the performance anxiety

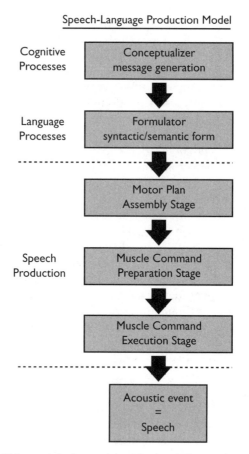

Speech-Language Production Model

Cognitive Processes — Conceptualizer message generation

Language Processes — Formulator syntactic/semantic form

Motor Plan Assembly Stage

Speech Production — Muscle Command Preparation Stage

Muscle Command Execution Stage

Acoustic event = Speech

FIGURE 5-3. This model of speech production helps students understand the rationale for relying on ideas rather than on specific words when making impromptu comments. From *Speaking: From Intention to Articulation*, p. 9, by W. J. M. Levelt, 1989, Cambridge: MIT Press. Copyright 1989 by MIT Press. Reprinted with permission.

suffered by famous people such as Streisand, Correlli, Olivier, and many sports figures is presented (See Chapter 1). The stories are reassuring to students, who begin to realize that their problem has little to do with skill or talent and that it is, in fact, a mind-body issue.

The first class ends with a final round of impromptu comments about ideas or insights that were particularly meaningful to individuals. This exercise reinforces the major points that were presented, elicits discussion and questions, and begins the desensitization to informal speaking in the group.

Homework Assignment

Assignments are then distributed for completion at home. Most important is the Personal Report of Communication Apprehension (PRCA 24) (McCroskey & Richmond, 1980, McCroskey, J. C., 2001), an instrument that measures the type and degree of communication apprehension in various situations (interpersonal, meetings, small groups, public speaking). Results help to provide students with a clearer understanding of where they stand on communication apprehension in relation to a general college population.

A fear hierarchy to guide students in their self-help program (Appendix 5-5) is then explained and distributed and a journal is assigned. Students are directed to record their reactions to the class and keep track of out-of-class assignments in the journal, enabling them to recognize changes in attitudes, behavior, and progress.

A bibliotherapy to supplement class work is also presented (See Suggested Readings). Entries marked with an asterisk are required student reading. Other references are recommended.

Class 2

Class 2 begins with a discussion of the reactions that were elicited by the homework questionnaires on the degree and types of communication apprehension (PRCA-24) and the hierarchies of speaking fears that they developed. Students are encouraged to begin gradually participating in feared situations outside of class and are reminded to record those events in their journals.

As discussed in Chapters 1 and 3, communication apprehension is further explained as a type of social anxiety leading to fear of formal and informal speaking situations, assertive interactions (talking to authorities, expressing disapproval of someone), and being observed. In its most severe form, social anxiety becomes a social phobia, in which there is a persistent fear of one or more situations when an individual is exposed to possible scrutiny by others. This fear results in people feeling that they may do something or act in a way that will be humiliating or embarrassing even though they recognize that their fear is excessive and unreasonable. Nevertheless, social and/or occupational functioning can be disrupted because of their avoidances or anxious endurance of common communicative situations. Students identify with this description of social phobia and find it extremely helpful as they begin to understand the problem and the universality of their fears.

Psychophysiology

The psychological explanation of social phobia culminates in an interactive lecture and slide presentation on the psychophysiology of performance anxiety, and the stress response. The presentation is aimed at diffusing the mythology of fear of speaking by explaining the problem physiologically and providing a basic understanding of the mind-body connection and the cognitive and self regulating strategies used to manage communication apprehension.

The slide presentation includes an overview of the nervous system, especially the branches of the autonomic nervous system (SNS and PNS) and the endocrine system (hypothalmic-pituitary axis). The differences between the sympathetic and parasympathetic systems, the effects of fear on stress hormone production, and the relationship of the respiratory and cardiovascular systems to hyperarousal and homeostasis are explained (See Chapters 2 and 4). Individual variations in reactivity, sympathetic/parasympathetic balance and response stereotypy are discussed. The power of the mind-body connection is emphasized. Examples of physiological changes that accompany a person's heightened emotions during stress, in some or all systems of the body are described. These include changes in breathing and heart rate, muscular tension, biochemistry, brain waves, temperature, and sweat gland responses. The mind-body connection is explained as an ancient concept that has been the basis for yoga and meditation techniques with specific types of breathing and postures to achieve calm states for thousands of years.

The difference between anxiety (subjective) and arousal (physiological) is clarified. As stated previously, anxiety is the subjective aspect of fear (real or perceived), and arousal is the physiological manifestation of anxiety. The importance of low, slow diaphragmatic breathing to reduce heart rate and other symptoms of hyperarousal is introduced.

Biofeedback   The effects of negative thinking and rapid and shallow breathing on hyperarousal are demonstrated clearly with the use of a handheld galvanic skin response (GSR) biofeedback instrument (See Figure 5-4). This instrument registers a high-pitched auditory signal when the body is under stress (e.g., with breath holding or tensed muscles) and provides a dramatic demonstration of the mind-body connection, especially for disbelievers.

The GSR actually measures variations in sweat gland activity and skin pore size, both controlled by the sympathetic nervous system. When excited, frightened, or disturbed to any degree, the body's system initiates chemical and physical changes throughout the organisms,

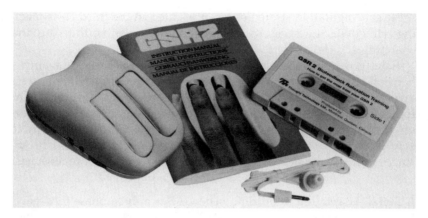

FIGURE 5-4. Handheld galvanic skin response (GSR) biofeedback device. Pictured is the GSR2. Photograph published with permission of Thought Technology, Montreal, Canada, *www.thought-technology.com*, 1-800-361-3651.

and the GSR level changes. These changes trigger the auditory signals of the GSR2 biofeedback device. Skin resistance increases when a person is calm and relaxed and decreases when a person is even slightly tense.

Fight or Flight The biofeedback demonstration is followed by an in-depth discussion of the significance of *interpretations* of events that either precipitate or ameliorate stress reactions. It is emphasized that it is the subjective view of an event, not the event itself, that triggers anticipatory anxiety and/or communication apprehension. This phenomenon is illustrated in the case example of Jose, who prepared well for his presentation, but fell apart when he noticed an audience member yawn as he spoke. He was so unnerved that he lost his train of thought and cut his interesting presentation short. In the debriefing following his presentation, the audience member who yawned explained that her reaction resulted from fatigue, not boredom or disinterest, as Jose had believed.

A discussion about of the pitfalls of faulty assumptions and (mis)interpretations of events inevitably leads to the importance of awareness about attitudes and thoughts that trigger the fight-or-flight response. Self-regulating strategies for gaining and maintaining control over stress reactions (hyperarousal), such as slow diaphragmatic breathing and progressive neuromuscular relaxation are introduced to reassure students that they can gain control over their physiological reactions to fear. More detailed explanations of these self-regulation strategies are presented in the third class meeting. However, the necessity for recognizing negative thinking and changing self-defeating thoughts is stressed.

Finally, the psychophysiological aspects of communication apprehension in relationship to the eustress, distress and optimal stress level phenomena which differs for each individual is discussed. The topics covered are (1) the point at which positive stress becomes negative, or distress; (2) homeostasis, the adaptive effort of the body to stay in balance; and (3) the general adaptation syndrome (GAS) stages of arousal that result from the effort to maintain homeostasis.

General Adaptation Syndrome   The GAS is a three-phase theoretical framework developed by the Canadian endocrinologist Hans Selye.[1] Although not specific, it was the first attempt to explain the human organism's effort to adapt physiologically to stress. Even though the GAS concept is considered simplistic today by physiologists (See Chapter 4), the author (B. H.) has found it useful in clarifying the mind-body connection and the etiology of the symptoms of stage fright. It is explained in the following way.

When an event is interpreted as a threat, the first phase of the GAS is initiated. The stressor causes a generalized somatic shock, or a call to arms, by the body's defense mechanisms which Cannon (1953) labeled the fight or flight reflex. These defense mechanisms include the endocrine system and the ANS adjustments. In the first phase, the endocrine axes, primarily the adrenal cortical system, are activated. The immediate result is an acceleration of the breathing rate (normally 12 to18 breaths per minute). The rapid, shallow breathing causes a person to exhale more carbon dioxide than normal. Because CO_2 is an acid, exhaling too much CO_2 leads to an imbalance in blood pH (the balance of acids and alkalis). If this condition persists, the body starts to react with a wide range of unpleasant sensations, a condition known as respiratory alkalosis, in which the endocrine system (especially the adrenal cortical system) is activated. As the body tries to restore balance, symptoms such as shortness of breath, tremors, weakness, chest pain, tingling, rapid heartbeat or palpitations, nausea, muscle shaking, and headache occur, making one feel as though they have lost control.

If the stress persists, the physiological responses of the alarm reaction diminish and the organism passes into the next phase of the GAS,

[1]Selye introduced contemporary notions about the relationship between stress and health. He noted that that the consequences of stress can be as harmful to health as a disease. Selye also noted that there are individual differences in the ability to cope with stressors, based on attitudes, perceptions, beliefs, and coping strategies, as well as genetic and acquired biological factors.

the state of resistance or adaptation, when localized somatic reactions such as breathing, heart rate, blood pressure, and temperature increase. This is when people usually say to themselves or others "calm down" or are enabled by the chemical changes in the nervous system to perform some emergency actions such as warding off attackers or chasing a thief. However, when someone is facing an audience, there is nobody to fight and nowhere to flee. Hence, the physiological reactions remain, even accelerate, with no release. If the stressor persists, eventually the "adaptive energy" involved in supporting this stage of resistance becomes depleted.

The organism then enters the third and final phase of the GAS, the stage of exhaustion. At this point, the body again triggers a generalized somatic alarm. The pituitary and adrenal cortex lose their ability to secrete hormones that resist stress, and the organism becomes defenseless. Continued stress at this level has even lead to death in some cases.

The maladaptive breathing symptoms, which begin in GAS stage 1 and escalate in stage 2 to hyperventilation (shallow irregular breathing, breath holding, sighing, tightness in the shoulders) actually exacerbate stress, sometimes leading to panic attacks unless brought under voluntary control.

Following the lecture and discussion about stress levels and the GAS, students (no exceptions) are called upon to address one or more points that had significance for them. They are free to remain seated or to stand. Their comments reinforce the information presented, continue the desensitization process of speaking in a group, and provide the basis for further discussions, questions, or insights.

The explanation of the cognitive and physiological symptoms of stage fright is highly effective in diffusing the mythologies about performance anxiety. Participants quickly realize that the stress response is the body's natural and adaptive way of reacting to a threatening event and that the mind makes no distinction between an actual and perceived threat. It also become clear that hyperarousal can be reduced through cognitive restructuring (recognizing and changing negative thoughts) and physiologically based relaxation techniques that restore autonomic nervous system balance (See Chapter 4). Finally, it is understood that the body's adaptive physiological reaction to challenge is nothing to be feared. The reaction must be recognized for what it is—priming the body for defensive action—something that can be a performer's best friend, if channeled correctly.

Model of Communication Apprehension: In an effort to integrate all of the essential information about communication apprehension, a model is presented. As shown in Figure 5-5, communication apprehension is

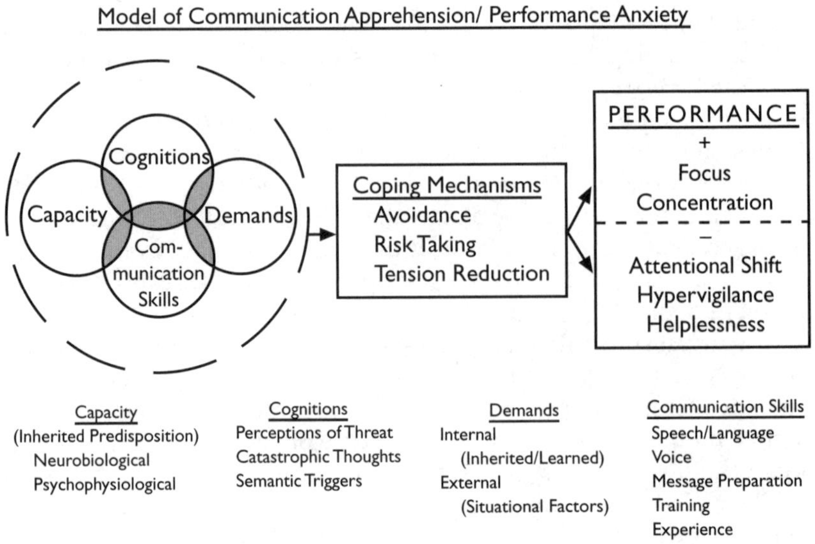

Model of Communication Apprehension/ Performance Anxiety

Capacity	Cognitions	Demands	Communication Skills
(Inherited Predisposition)	Perceptions of Threat	Internal	Speech/Language
Neurobiological	Catastrophic Thoughts	(Inherited/Learned)	Voice
Psychophysiological	Semantic Triggers	External	Message Preparation
		(Situational Factors)	Training
			Experience

FIGURE 5-5. Cognition, demand, capacity, and skill level combine to evoke communication apprehension/performance anxiety and lead to reaction by coping mechanisms, resulting in both positive (+) and negative (−) aspects of performance.

viewed as a capacity-demands model. Capacity is an individual's pre-disposition to be aroused, based on psychophysiological and neurobiological factors. Demands include external (real) and internal (imagined) stress factors. The cognitive component is how one interprets a stimulus and whether or not thoughts take over the body. The skills component is the integrity of the speech/motor system and linguistic competence (knowledge) and performance coupled with training and experience.

With the exception of innate neurobiological and psychophysiological elements, the negative components of the model can be reduced and the positive components reinforced through insight and training. Even the capacity element can be modified in some individuals with intensive, early intervention, or through medication.

Treatment of communication apprehension in the Speaking Without Fear class is based on the above model and includes cognitive/behavioral, physiological, affective, and experiential targets, as well as enhancement of communication skills.

Communication apprehension is then viewed from the perspective of possible predisposing, precipitating, and perpetuating causes leading to the fear of speaking. The facilitator discusses the three perspectives illustrated with case examples and encourages comments from group members who can identify with the situations presented. This discussion is often provocative for students who frequently recall events in their background that might have contributed to their problems.

Discussion: Factors Related to Communication Apprehension

Predisposing Factors   Predisposing factors for performance anxiety are discussed, using anonymous case examples of previous students. Group members are encouraged to talk about their own experiences. Topics include excessive reticence in early childhood that may persist into adulthood and hypervigilance to internal bodily reactions ("I've always been that way"). In addition, the discussion covers traits such as perfectionism, unrealistic personal standards, and personalities who rely on others for a sense of worth, as well as overly sensitive persons who are at high risk for threat perception. Learned factors such as nonassertiveness, unconscious cultural hooks of strict inhibitions against emotional displays, gender and social rules (who speaks to whom and how), unconscious personal hooks that cause an inordinate fear of criticism ("I must not") or a lack of modeling ("I don't know how") are also presented. Finally, the innate fear of visual scrutiny that leads one to associate being looked at and being the center of attention with fear of attack is discussed. Students are generally very relieved following the discussion of predisposing factors because they realize, often for the first time, that they are not weak, sick, crazy, or unique. They frequently express comfort in knowing that there are rational reasons for their seemingly irrational fears.

Precipitating Factors   Precipitating fears of communication are explored through a discussion of examples of early traumatic events related to performing and/or communicating. Precipitators include such factors as audience size, composition, or hostility, cognitive dissonance (speaking about things that conflict with basic values), inexperience, inadequate preparation, or overpreparation (excessive information or broad topics).

Perpetuating Factors   Discussion of factors that perpetuate communication apprehension includes misinformation about performance anxiety ("What is it?" "Why me?"), misperceptions of self by self and others ("my fears are visible; everyone is okay but me"), habituated negative coping strategies ("if I don't talk, they won't know how frightened I am; if I talk they will know how **+# I am"), fear of being oneself (trying to impress rather than express), and the cycle of fear which involves arousal→subjective interpretations (misinterpretations of fear)→hypervigilance→attentional shifts→catastrophic thoughts→lack of focus→poor performance→negative expectations→avoidance/panic.

Class 2 usually ends on an upbeat note because many misconceptions about communication apprehension have been clarified. The following comments from a final round of impromptu presentations are typical of students' reactions to this class.

- "It makes me feel better to know that others share the same feelings."
- "It is a relief to know that there is a name, that it is a universal problem, and what it is."
- "I take comfort in understanding the way the body works and that it can be balanced."
- "I like the sense of control that we can get by effectively dealing with the body's adrenaline release."
- "I learned how important your thoughts are and that you must correct your negative thinking."
- "It is the first time I heard that my reactions are a result of the way I think."
- "The reasoning behind the fear ... there's hope through relaxed, correct breathing."
- "I feel enlightened. We discussed so many variables and tools. ... it's comforting."
- "This has been an extensive trip, I had no idea ... I wasn't aware of any of this. I'm overwhelmed and so excited, it's so important for me... I have so many ideas and I just can't say them to the people who matter."
- "I never thought about the messages I received as a kid. ... wow, they can be loaded."

Homework Assignment

Students are given a homework assignment to reflect about their formative years to determine how the early messages they received pertain to their adult attitudes and a "What if?" exercise (Appendix 5-3) that helps them separate fantasy fears from reality-based fears. They are also given a Psychophysiological Diary form on which to note events that trigger negative thoughts resulting in stress symptoms (Appendix 5-4).

Class 3

There are three goals in the third class meeting: (1) to disseminate and discuss personality test results that inform individuals about innate and learned behaviors that contribute to their performance anxiety, (2) to present several self-regulation strategies for control of mental and physio-logical arousal related to feared performances, and (3) to provide infor-mation about the development and delivery of oral presentations.

The class opens with a discussion of progress noted by students during the preceding week. Someone invariably reports a dramatic breakthrough, primarily because he or she understood, for the first time, the bases of their fears and/or implemented some suggestion offered casually during the first two classes. It is not uncommon to hear "it's a miracle. ... for the first time I ..." This sharing time is important for facilitating spontaneous speaking in the group, height-ening the group's cohesiveness, evoking insights and associations, and encouraging all to take risks.

Results of the personality tests taken during the first class are dis-tributed. Students are informed about their risk tendencies for threat perception (Wickramasekera, 1998). Some classic reactions to these test results have been:

- "I always knew I was sensitive but not to that degree."
- "Now I understand why I start off okay, but then panic in the middle of a presentation."
- "Now I understand the disconnection between my mind and body. ... It's okay to be sensitive. It's a strength, not a weakness, but I must learn to toughen up and not react to what I think others are thinking of me."

Further inquiry about the implications of the tests often results in con-tinued therapy after the completion of the course, as the information provokes considerable thought and profound insights that can lead to remarkable breakthroughs in communication apprehension.

Cognitive Awareness Exercises

After review of the Psychophysiological Diary (homework assign-ment), in which students recorded their automatic negative thoughts about an upsetting communication incident, several activities that focus on awareness and the restructuring of negative thoughts that are at the core of communication apprehension are presented. The development of hyperarousal and the negative cycle of fear of perfor-mance becomes clear, as the relationship of a feared event, negative thinking, and physical symptoms is traced. Ways of defusing fears by reformulating negative thoughts into positive coping statements are demonstrated. Some examples of these cognitive changes are:

Negative Automatic Thoughts	Reformulated Positive Thoughts
"They will think I am stupid."	"I am actually reasonably intelligent."
"I will say nothing worthwhile."	"I have some good ideas."
"I can't make a mistake."	"It's okay to make a mistake."
"I'm going to faint."	"My breathing makes me feel dizzy."

In a small group exercise, students restructure each others' negative statements. One student from each group reports to the class on their most effective reformulations. This exercise is followed by some examples of commonly distorted cognitions. These include:

- **Filtering:** You take negative details and magnify them while filtering out all positive aspects of a situation.
- **Polarized thinking:** Things are either good or bad, there is no middle ground. You have to be perfect or you are a failure.
- **Mind reading:** You are positive that you know what others are thinking about your performance and why they behave as they do.
- **Overgeneralizing:** You come to a general conclusion based on a single incident or piece of evidence. If you forgot a line or had a problem once, you fully expect it to happen repeatedly. "I always ..."
- **Catastrophizing:** You expect disaster. You notice something and obsess with "what ifs."
- **Emotional reasoning:** You believe that what you feel must be true automatically. If you feel stupid and boring, then you must be stupid and boring.
- **Should statements:** You have a list of ironclad rules about how you should speak or perform and feel guilty if you don't live up to them (e.g., "I should have said it that way.")

Participants are encouraged to help each other refute unrealistic, negative, or distorted thoughts when comments on feelings about class performances are elicited. Everyone benefits by this open exchange of feedback, as students quickly recognize the distorted self-perceptions of others.

"What If?" Exercise

The "What if?" exercise is then reviewed. This homework assignment (See Appendix 5-3) is particularly effective in (objectively) crystallizing the absurdity of communication apprehension. Students conjure up an imagined fearful event and record what negative reaction can possibly occur if they engage in the event. They continue the "What if?" exercise to the point of absurdity. They can reverse this exercise by approaching their reactions positively. Amazing things happen when paper tiger fears are directly confronted. Generally, the consequences of imagined fears are so outrageous that they loose their impact when carefully analyzed. A negative "what if?" scenario might (be):

> "What if I can't think of anything to say? *Then, I won't be asked to come back again.* And if I'm not asked to come back again? *They will never know how to do xyz.* And if they don't know how to do xyz? *They will have to ask me how to do it.* And if they ask me how to do it? *They will have to ask me to come back!"*

Physiological Strategies

Quieting Response One of the most effective strategies for fast-acting relief from stressful reactions is the quieting response, popularized by Dr. Chuck Stroeble. If done correctly, this brief breathing exercise offers a quick way to calm down through several rounds of correct "low/slow" diaphragmatic breaths that result in a deceleration of heart rate, and even negative thoughts. The instructions (Girdano & Everly, 1980) are:

1. Assume a comfortable position, resting the left hand, palm down, on the navel, with the right hand over the left. Eyes should be closed to eliminate distractions.
2. Recognize the direction of abdominal movement during inhalation (abdomen should expand) and exhalation (abdomen should recede) as the lungs fill up with air and release CO_2.
3. Imagine a hollow bottle lying internally beneath the hands as you inhale. Take in the air through your nose (do not work at inhaling), feeling the air descend slowly to the pouch. The total length of the inhalation should be 2 seconds.
4. Hold the breath "in the pouch" for 2 seconds, repeating the phrase, "my body is calm."
5. Slowly begin to exhale; emptying the pouch while repeating to yourself, "my body is calm." The exhalation should be two or three times [longer than] the inhalation. (Remember, that as one inhales the heart rate accelerates, and during exhalation it decelerates. The object of this exercise is to slow the heart rate, which will, in turn, reduce the cascade of stress hormones from the brain-B.H.).

6. Repeat this exercise three to five times in succession. If you feel light-headedness—stop. If lightheadedness recurs with continued practice, simply shorten the length of the inhalation and/or decrease the number of times you repeat the exercise.

This brief exercise should be practiced 20–40 times a day in order to develop the ability to temporarily relax "on the spot" in anxiety-producing situations. Consistent practice can lead to a more relaxed and calmer attitude—a sort of antistress attitude—and will be helpful in lessening symptoms during stressful moments. It also helps people recognize their tendencies for breath holding and irregular breathing during anxious moments. This is important, because hyperventilation escalates hyperarousal in addition to contributing to its cause in a chicken-and-egg cycle. Breath holding must be quickly identified and released, because it can trigger panic if continued for longer than 17 seconds (Fried, 1990).

The handheld GSR 2, discussed earlier, is again used to demonstrate the effects of correct low/slow diaphragmatic breathing on the autonomic nervous system. The auditory signal from the instrument, which increases in pitch and intensity with arousal and disappears with relaxation, is dramatic evidence of how this type of breathing can reduce hyperarousal. Students invariably report that they feel calm and relaxed after a few rounds of the quieting response exercise.

Heart Rate Training A program for systematically training individuals in diaphragmatic breathing to reduce anxiety in patients with anxiety disorders, asthma and stuttering as well as to optimize performance of all sorts has been developed in Russia. A portable biofeedback instrument called a cardiosignalizer is used to track the synchrony between breathing and heart rate and measures respiratory sinus arrhythmia (RSA) (See Chapter 4). It is claimed that when synchrony is achieved with intensive training, RSA is maximized, resulting in the establishment of homeostasis, a balance between the sympathetic and parasympathetic nervous systems. As mentioned previously, it is the imbalance of the ANS that is considered to be the physiological basis of anxiety.

The use of the cardiosignalizer for heart rate training through correct diaphragmatic breathing has been demonstrated in class and has been used selectively with a few individual clients who reported improvement. The author (BH) looks forward to the results of research on RSA training with heart rate instrumentation which is now ongoing with asthmatic patients (See Recent Advances, this chapter), as it holds promise for a more systematic and rapid reduction of anxiety for communication apprehension as well.

However, at present more traditional relaxation exercises for anxiety reduction are demonstrated in class for practice at home. These include progressive neuromuscular relaxation, centering activities, autogenic training, self-talk, visual imagery, physiological quieting responses (respiratory), assertiveness strategies and diet control.

Neuromuscular Relaxation Exercise To create awareness of bodily tensions, Jacobson's progressive relaxation exercise is demonstrated (Jacobson, 1974). This exercise requires participants to tense each set of muscles twice for about 5 seconds beginning with the toes and gradually working up the entire body. Students are instructed to breathe normally during muscular contractions or to inhale as they tense and exhale as they release tension. If done correctly, this exercise should take about 20 minutes to relax the entire body. It takes less time for only a few muscle groups. It should be practiced at home and used before stressful speaking situations to reduce muscle tension. Students are also encouraged to do frequent body scans to determine sites of muscle tension and to release it. This exercise is effective in raising awareness of muscle tension without biofeedback equipment that records and reflects states of tension.

Centering Centering is a concept taken from Buddhism that refers to *chi*, *qi*, or *ki*, the life force. According to tradition, one's center is 2 inches below one's navel and 2 inches into the body. Centering techniques are helpful in achieving focus. One technique used in class has three steps involving three breaths with three different mental processes (Greene, 1998). The instructions are:

1. With the first breath, on the inhalation, think only about a full and deep breath. Inhale slowly through the nose, paying full attention to the breath. As you slowly exhale, release all of the muscle tension, in the arms, shoulders, and neck. Feel heavy or loose, releasing all of your tensions.
2. On the second breath, be at your center, 2 inches below your navel and 2 inches into your body toward your backbone. Put your hand there and try to bring your mind there. Get out of your head into your center.
3. On the third breath, as you inhale, think a positive word or phrase that is descriptive of your ability to express yourself at your best. (e.g., "warm, calm, safe, confident"). Do this as you inhale and begin to exhale. While you are doing this, either look at a nondescript spot on the floor, blur your focus, or close your eyes, remaining inward.

As you complete your exhalation turn your focus or energy out, directing your full attention to a specific point in the group, directing your energy or ki outward.

Students are told to practice this exercise several times whenever they feel anxious about performing. In addition, they are urged to "center" while imagining participation in a difficult meeting or other stressful speaking situations. The process allows one to gain self-control and enables focusing in a threatening situation.

There are two other centering activities that are used to help students control their mental fears. The first one involves closing the eyes and focusing only on the breath during inhalation and exhalation, but acknowledging and then letting go of intrusive thoughts by returning back to focus on the breath. The other centering activity involves playing mentally with the sounds in the environment, at first straining to hear everything (a narrow focus) and then reversing the mental set and just letting the sounds come (an open focus). Students are encouraged to recognize the difference in the two mental states, trying and just being, and to learn to let go of intrusive or obsessive thoughts which disrupt concentration.

Autogenic Training (self-regulation) Thermal regulation is directly connected to the sympathetic nervous system and is a sensitive and widely used measure of arousal and control. For many people hand temperature is low during states of arousal. To reduce hyperarousal or excessive sympathetic nervous system activity, a type of self-hypnosis, autogenic training, is discussed and demonstrated with the use of a small finger thermometer taped to the finger. This exercise helps students learn about their ability to self-regulate the physiological process of thermal control by observing increases in their hand temperature resulting from mental recitation of a script that emphasizes relaxation and warmth.

Self-Talk Another effective way of dealing with intrusive, negative thoughts that creep into the mind during centering exercises is to name the fears, which are referred to as gremlins. Once they are named, the gremlins are mentally told to "get lost". Interestingly, one student called her gremlin "grandma" because her grandmother, who raised her and whom she could never please, was a cold, overburdened woman who did nothing to nurture or encourage her. Another student named her gremlin Larry, the name of her third grade classmate in a new school who tormented her about her ethnicity and size until she was fearful of speaking to anyone. She never told anyone about Larry and harbored her gremlin, who continued to torment her for 20 years before exposing him in a place where she felt safe, the class. Anthropomorphizing their paper tiger gremlins enabled both of these students to gain some insight into the source of their fears as well as feel a sense of power over some old, lethal ghosts.

Two other powerful self-talk strategies for stopping ruminations about negativity are presented. Students are instructed to tell themselves to STOP, LET IT GO, while snapping a thick rubber band worn on their wrist. Another suggestion is to tell students to float with their anxiety, not to fight it, while realizing that it won't harm them. (See Floating in Chapter 3). In addition, powerful guided visual imagery exercises are used to change negative thinking and fearful images.

Guided Visualization/Imagery Desensitization Imagery is a basic medium of the unconscious mind along with emotional feelings and kinesthetic sensations. Guided imagery is a method of deliberately using visualization to modify thinking, feeling (physiological and emotional), and behavior that has been used to modify behavior in profound ways. It has successfully reversed a variety of diseases including cancer as well as helped in overcoming phobias. This has been accomplished by techniques which guide visualizations of internal warriors that fight disease processes and/or fears. Visual imagery is also widely used by professional athletes to achieve peak or optimal performances.

The guided imagery exercise for overcoming communication apprehension begins with a centering technique that employs diaphragmatic breathing while sitting comfortably in a quiet location. Students are instructed to close their eyes and to think of a place that is especially peaceful for them, a beach, a lake, or the mountains. This should be any place where they can get in touch with all of their senses: temperature, touch, sight, smell, and hearing. Once they arrive at a state of complete calm, they are instructed to imagine, in their mind's eye, going through a presentation from beginning to end as they continue being centered and breathing slowly. They are instructed to visualize the designated room or hall and the audience, hear their introduction, present their complete message, and imagine the applause and/or accolades afterward for a job well done. Positive key words or phrases that they associate with the event should be selected prior to the visualization and be incorporated with their image. Such words as "warm and safe" or "express and converse" have been effective verbal images for students who thought carefully about times when they performed well. Students are encouraged to focus on these words and to use them as a mantra for all speaking situations that they encounter. It may be necessary to change the key words at a later time if the phrase loses effectiveness or if the situation changes significantly.

Calming scenes should be tape recorded by the student or a friend (with a pleasant voice) and listened to regularly at home while imaging a particular performance situation. The imagery should be combined with a complete state of relaxation and positive words. It is especially important that students consider the imagery desensitization technique a necessary part of their preparation and rehearsal time, for visual imagery and silent rehearsal are powerful techniques to achieve peak performance.

Assertiveness Techniques

Little time is scheduled for assertiveness techniques in the group, although this is often a major need for some students, particularly those from cultures or backgrounds that admonish children for being outspoken or expressing feelings, especially in public. When it is apparent that cultural hooks or personality styles (learned or genetic) are the bases for inordinate speaking fears, students are helped to recognize their underlying conflicts and encouraged to express their opinions, talk about their feelings, to say "no" (and mean it), and to resolve conflicts in a direct, diplomatic way that is not confrontational (leveling). This later involves learning to say: "I know … I feel … why I feel … I want … can we reach an understanding or work this out?" The group can be very effective in encouraging nonassertive students to speak up and speak out, sometimes for the first time. Once the ice is broken, the previously nonassertive students begin taking more risks and usually make good progress. At the very least they begin to recognize the existence and effects of their nonassertiveness and are encouraged to seek professional help to overcome their problem.

Lifestyle/Nutrition

Nutrition is discussed because diet is related to stress and anxiety. It has been well documented that certain foods and substances create additional stress and anxiety, while others promote a calming effect (Bourne, 1995). Students are cautioned about overuse of stimulants such as caffeine, which can aggravate or create stress. Caffeine is known as a sympathomimetic substance that mimics the effects of the sympathetic nervous system. It increases the level of the neurotransmitter norepinephrine in the brain, leading to a feeling of alertness—also producing the very same physiological arousal response that is triggered by stress. That is, there is an increase in sympathetic nervous system activity and a release of adrenaline. Caffeine is found not only in coffee, but also in many types of tea, cola beverages, chocolate candy, cocoa, and over-the-counter drugs. Although there are individual differences in caffeine sensitivity, students who are prone to generalized anxiety or panic attacks, are advised to reduce their consumption to less than 100 mg/day (one 6-oz cup of coffee). Nicotine is as strong a stimulant as caffeine and is also discouraged. In general, a wholesome lifestyle that includes healthy diet, exercise, and sleep are recommended to enhance coping with performance anxiety. There is no place for all-nighters, excessive caffeine intake, smoking, and unhealthy lifestyles, if someone is serious about overcoming communication apprehension.

Johari Window

A brief explanation of our many selves (public, private, blind, and closed) is presented to inform people that we do not see ourselves as others see us (See Chapter 2 for discussion of the Johari Window). This concept is helpful in reinforcing the notion that individuals are generally not good judges of their own performances and should rely on the feedback of others, as well as on objectively viewing their own video-tapes, to readjust their self-perceptions.   .

Impromptu Presentations

Volunteers are solicited to comment on information or strategies presented in class that were particularly meaningful to them. However, this time they are encouraged to leave their seats and speak in front of the group. Students usually begin implementing some of the techniques discussed earlier (e.g., quieting response or imagery), as they cope with what has become known as the "creeping death syndrome" (waiting your turn to speak). This round of presentations is a way of reinforcing and clarifying the information presented earlier. All group members are required to say something, even if they are not yet ready to leave their seats. There is then a 10-minute break.

Anatomy of a Presentation

Following the break, the remainder of the class addresses ways to develop the four modes of oral presentations: impromptu, interactive, extemporaneous, and manuscript. The particular mode used depends on the structure or formality of a situation. Impromptu and interactive presentations require little planning. Extemporaneous and manuscript presentations require extensive preparation and rehearsal. Students will have already engaged in several impromptu and interactive presentations in class.

Types of Presentations

Impromptu An impromptu presentation is a spontaneous, informal talk, usually no longer than 2 minutes that is often used when reporting or explaining something. Suggestions for developing an impromptu presentation include formulating a central idea, agreeing or disagreeing with a previous speaker, using one of the five Ws (who, what where, when, and how) or the PREP formula (P = point, R = reason, E = example, P = point reiterated). The PREP formula provides a structure to organize, plan, and make a point. Students are provided frequent opportunities to make impromptu presentations in class and encouraged to do so whenever possible on their jobs or in their communities.

Interactive Interactive presentations involve a question-answer exchange. It usually starts with an impromptu presentation establishing rapport with the audience, followed by questions from the audience. Hence, interactive presentations mimic or become a conversation that is easier to manage than a more formal presentation.

Extemporaneous/Manuscript Extemporaneous presentations are the most frequent type of speech for formal situations and require planning, development, and rehearsal. Having a definite purpose, format, and organizational framework, they are delivered from notes and can be punctuated with visual aids. The format includes an introduction, body, and conclusion.

The next task for students is to prepare such a presentation. The steps they are to follow are:

- Select a manageable topic suitable for a specified time frame and establish the purpose of the presentation (informative, persuasive, inspirational, or special occasion).
- Analyze the audience in terms of demographics, opinion leaders, beliefs, attitudes and values, and knowledge of the topic.
- Research the topic and develop such supporting evidence as statistics, examples, experiences, expert testimony, and useful analogies.
- Organize the materials logically, including an effective introduction, anecdotes and interesting details (hooks), body, and conclusion.
- Develop notes for delivery (cards, overheads, flip charts, visual aids).
- Anticipate questions and answers.
- Rehearse with a friend, tape recorder, or video camera.
- Use desensitizing imagery to alleviate and prevent fears.

Manuscript presentations are simply elaborated extemporaneous presentations in which the entire speech is written. They are generally appropriate for formal occasions such as after-dinner speeches or official talks that are to be recorded or published. Students are referred to a speech communication text for further reading on the preparation of extemporaneous and manuscript presentations. However, the major emphasis is on how to prepare and rehearse well—for lack of adequate preparation is preparation for hyperarousal.

Delivery Hints

Students are encouraged to think of the delivery of their well-prepared, visualized, and rehearsed presentations as enlarged conversations. They are motivated to express, not impress; to be themselves, their best selves; to get centered and focused; and to use all the strategies that work for them to control their fears. They are also warned to expect some arousal before they present, especially when speaking to a group has been scrupulously avoided for a long time, and to channel the arousal into constructive energy and expression. Students are also reminded to eliminate negative ruminations and distorted thoughts that may occur and to think positively, using their selected positive mantras. They are also reminded to do centering and imaging exercises in preparation for their presentations and to repeat the processes immediately before they present. No further instructions about delivery are given during this class.

Homework

The assignment for the next class meeting is then given. It is a short (7-minute) demonstration, a how-to talk that will teach the group some activity that each presenter enjoys doing. Two minutes are to be allotted for questions. The talk can be on a hobby-, sport-, or work-related topic and speakers can determine who the audience should be. Students are encouraged to use props or visuals for overhead projection, or to engage the audience in a simple activity. They are reminded to have their own VHS tapes for videotaping the following week and to continue their journals and stress-reducing activities at home. Class 3 usually ends with trepidation, as students are challenged by what seems to be an enormous undertaking: choosing a topic and (preparing) the following week's speech assignment.

Class 4

At the beginning of Class 4, students are requested to speak to their neighbor about their presentation, because they will introduce each other. This tactic seems to reduce the tension and enables students to speak twice in one evening. Each speaker is allotted 10 to 12 minutes, depending on the size of the group. One person is appointed as time-keeper and gives the speaker a hand or written sign indicating that they have 2 minutes to wrap up and/or entertain questions. A videographer tapes the speakers, who are introduced by their neighbors. Each speaker is asked to comment on how he or she feels following the presentation and to rate his or her performance before feedback is elicited from the audience.

As each class is composed of an interesting and diversified group of people, the presentations are generally fun and received with spontaneous applause. Little evidence of nervousness is apparent to the audience, although speakers are consistently convinced that their anxiety was evi-dent to everyone. Feedback from the audience usually refutes any misper-ceptions that the speaker had about his or her performance and is generally honest and supportive. The facilitator comments only after the general audience reacts. It is only at this time that suggestions on delivery or speech/voice issues are addressed. Other reactions and comments not previously covered are also given, usually in the form of leading questions (e.g., How many times did you practice the presentation? What happened when? etc.). Speakers are then given a form and asked to rate their level of fear and mental and physical reactions to compare with their previous pre-sentations. Videotapes are returned to the students for home viewing.

Homework

Assignments for the following four classes are given. Students are to prepare two informative presentations, one persuasive or motivational presentation, or an oral reading (some students fear reading more than speaking for a variety of personal reasons). These talks will gradually increase in length, depending on the size of the class, with time always allotted for questions. If desired, the topics can be work-related, and speakers can request that the group role play a target audience for them (e.g., jury, hostile managers).

Class 5

Class 5 begins with a discussion of reactions to the videotapes of the previous class which were viewed at home. There is generally unanim-ity in reactions about the viewings, as people are amazed that they came across so well, with no evidence of the anxiety they were certain was visible to all. The taped visual feedback is powerful in dispelling unrealistic self-perceptions about the ability to speak in front of a group, resulting in a major boost in confidence and self-esteem.

Students also report on progress that they made or problems that they encountered during the week.

The fifth class generally runs very smoothly, because the audience becomes so involved in the array of interesting topics presented that some people forget the reasons they enrolled in the class in the first place. Nevertheless, the audience and the facilitator, who is continually amazed at the rapid progress in attitudes and performances made in such a short time, give verbal feedback to each speaker. Specific suggestions regarding preparation, content, delivery, and anxiety reduction strategies are offered, as needed.

Classes 6 and 7

The format of Classes 6 and 7 is the same as that of the previous ones with a few notable exceptions. Visitors are invited to attend, and the length of presentations is increased, when possible. Based on the number of students and the classroom arrangement, variables are introduced to reduce the adaptation effect and increase external stress. This is helpful in promoting generalization to situations outside of the classroom. As always, reactions to previous tapings and progress in the real world are discussed. Then, students are introduced for the next round of videotaped presentations. But at these times, students are challenged by the audience, who have been prompted to feign hostility or ignorance. Speakers are expected to defuse these situations tactfully. Presentations are then critiqued. By the later classes, students who have become extremely perceptive in recognizing and refuting spurious or negative thinking often preempt the facilitator's comments.

Class 8

The final class differs only in its ambiance, because it is a celebration. Everyone contributes food or drink for an informal buffet, and students become after-dinner speakers. The same format used in the previous classes is followed. However, this time students are requested to rate their fears and draw them as they did during the first class. The sketches, albeit simplistic, are powerful evidence of the mind-body connection. Comparisons of drawings at the end of the course with the initial sketches from the first class tangibly demonstrates to students the extent of their progress in reducing phobic attitudes to speaking situations and overcoming their communication apprehension.

In a final round of impromptu presentations, students are asked to react to the entire program and to complete a form about how their anxiety about speaking in public changed as part of their experience.

All students are encouraged to follow up the introductory Speaking Without Fear class by enrolling in other speaking or performance courses, the monthly booster session offered by the instructor, of Toastmasters International, or to start their own speaking groups on the job. Some students choose to continue on a private basis or are referred to specific specialists, such as speech or voice therapists or psychotherapists, if necessary. Most students feel that they have made sufficient progress to continue successfully on their own.

For many students, the class serves not only as an opportunity for overcoming speaking fears, but also as a social and professional networking opportunity. All generally acknowledge the class as a positive and productive experience. For some, it has proven to be a life-altering experience, something they never anticipated could happen in so short a time.

Treatment Issues for Other Communication Disorders

In addition to communication apprehension, some voice and speech problems can also be somatizations of unconscious fears. As SLPs generally have not been educated or trained to consider the mind-body connection in their clinical work, patients with questionable or seemingly intangible complaints may be considered uncooperative or unmanageable. In cases of intransigent dysphonias, behavioral approaches (masking, cough extension, or inhalation phonation), digital manipulation or botulinum injections are generally used to reduce the symptoms, while other behavioral approaches have been employed with recalcitrant speech disorders (e.g., persistent lisps or dysfluencies). However, these approaches seldom uncover or address the source of a problem, which even if relieved, can recur, depending on the persistence of the unconscious fears. Understanding the mind-body connection is vital for speech clinicians who often confront problems caused or exacerbated by unconscious anxiety. Therefore, it is important for SLPs to understand how anxiety can be objectively measured with biofeedback equipment such as electromyography (EMG), electroencelography (EEG), thermal (temperature variation), and galvanic skin response (GSR) devices, respirotracers, and heart rate trackers (cardiosignalizers).

Anxiety Reduction for Speech/Voice Problems

In treating speech and voice problems of unknown etiology and possible psychological origin, Wickramasekera's High Risk Model of Threat Perception (1999) is helpful. As discussed in Chapter 2, Wickramasekera hypothesized that high and low hypnotic ability in interaction with negative affect contributes to the production and reduction of clinical symptoms. He postulates that this happens because high and low hypnotizability is related to the dysregulation of the sympathetic and parasympathetic branches of the autonomic nervous system. Wickramasekera states that biofeedback is most effective for reducing clinical symptoms in people of low to moderate hypnotic ability, while training in self-hypnosis or other instructional procedures such as autogenic training, progressive muscle regulation and/or meditation with cognitive behavioral therapy will produce the most rapid reduction of clinical symptoms with people high in trait hypnotic ability. These two approaches to anxiety reduction and symptom relief are described as top-down and bottom-up and are selected on the basis of patients' personality profiles and reactions to stress.

Top-Down Approach   The top-down approach in reducing anxiety is suggested for individuals with high trait hypnotic ability, that is, those in touch with their physiological and emotional feelings even though they may not understand the mind-body connection. It begins by helping clients acknowledge and restructure their thoughts and attitudes, and includes self-regulation techniques, progressive muscle regulation relaxation, mediation, and cognitive-behavioral techniques. This is the approach used in the Speaking Without Fear course.

The author (B. H.) also found the top-down approach also effective with a variety of other anxiety-related communication disorders when clients were aware of their feelings, had a trusting relationship with the clinician, and a desire to change. (See the case examples of language, speech, and voice disorders in Chapters 1 and 2.)

Bottom-Up Approach   The bottom-up approach in reducing anxiety is recommended for individuals who are not in touch with their emotions—that is, those with low to moderate hypnotic trait ability. This approach begins by showing individuals how their body systems respond on biofeedback instruments. The physiological findings are powerful evidence of the consequences of repressed emotions and are effective in helping these clients acknowledge the source of their problems and how they *really* feel and react to stress.

People who deny having anxiety or worry, often become sick with common somatic complaints that are related to psychosocial problems such as fears about being assertive, socializing, expressing feelings, and communicating. This patient population has been identified in busy voice and speech clinics (Hickman, personal communication).

Wickramasekera postulates that people with low hypnotic ability unconsciously keep their stress a secret from their conscious mind but not from their body, which reacts to the stress. This response is typical of those who are unable to discuss feelings and/or moods, a condition known as alexythymia. Such patients are very concrete and tend to attribute psychological changes to external stimuli (the weather or food) or speak of psychological states (depression) in somatic language such as pain (Sifneos, 1972, Wickramasekera, 1998).

A Trojan horse approach has been successfully used to convince patients who do not believe that memories and beliefs have biological consequences that their symptoms are related to anxiety. First, physiological responses to neutral and emotional material presented by the clinician are measured with biofeedback instrumentation. When patients are shown their heightened physiological responses to emotional material, they are able to recognize connections between what they think and feel and their physical symptoms. Only then are they able to address their toxic issues. This insight serves as the beginning of relief from such typical somatic symptoms as muscle tensions, pain, respiratory distress, and elevated blood pressure.

The use of biofeedback instrumentation is an essential and effective part of the bottom-up approach. This is because instrumentation can detect tiny signals of tension or anxiety that an individual may deny or not be able to recognize until it is greatly intensified and more difficult to control. EMG has already been used by some speech-language pathologists and biofeedback clinicians with voice disorders with success (Davids, Smith, & Montgomery, 1996; Sime & Healey, 1993). EMG biofeedback has also been used successfully in a public speaking workshop (Hickerson & Shannon, 1998). As mentioned previously, this author (B. H.) has used digital thermometers and a handheld GSR instrument for demonstration and therapy with clients otherwise not aware of how their thoughts influenced their arousal and subsequent speaking and singing performances.

Example: The $2 Million Man

Wickramasekera has described a patient with a host of serious physical problems who underwent a $2 million medical workup, which was unsuccessful in determining a diagnosis, all paid for by his insurance companies. The man's condition remained undiagnosed until he was referred, as a last resort, to a physiological psychologist, (Dr. Wickramasekera).

Initially the patient denied any unhappiness other than his serious medical conditions. However, it wasn't until a psychophysiological profile was performed that the source of his illness was determined: his intensely negative feelings about his wife and marriage, a secret he had locked up in his unconscious. Only after he recognized the problem with the help of biofeedback-generated physiological measurements (e.g., skyrocketing blood pressure and other measures only when he talked to or about his wife), acknowledged its source, and worked it through verbally, did his symptoms disappear. His medical conditions had been somatizations of his overwhelming, unconscious negative feelings about his marriage and sexual identity, problems of which he had been completely unaware. This serious medical problem was resolved very quickly in a few sessions with an integrated psychophysiological and cognitive approach to therapy.

This dramatic case suggests that the most efficacious way to treat somatized anxiety symptoms with people who repress their feelings is with psychophysiological profiling and biofeedback integrated with talk therapy.

Implications for Speech-Language Pathology

The $2 million man case illustrates the importance of the ability to recognize and acknowledge feelings in every field of health care. This is especially so in speech-language pathology for several reasons. First, the laryngeal system is part of the respiratory system, the primary purpose of which is to sustain life. Voice and speech are overlaid functions of this survival mechanism. When the respiratory system is disturbed by anxiety or intense emotions, allergic and asthmatic reactions are exacerbated. Interestingly, children who stutter have been found to have more problems with asthma, allergies, and upper respiratory distress than children who do not stutter. Consequently, those who stutter have more difficulty speaking during states of arousal (Freeman, personal communication, 1998). Moreover, according to Bless, Swift, Swift, Pasic, and Sandage (1999) 50% of patients with paradoxical vocal fold dysfunction have been diagnosed (or misdiagnosed) with asthma suggesting an underlying or exacerbating emotional component in some cases. Finally, the author (B. H.) has noted a preponderance of histories of allergies and asthma in families of participants enrolled in the classes of Speaking Without Fear.

It is clear that emotions influence highly sensitive airways, which in turn affect voice and speech production. For this reason alone, it is important that speech-language pathologists understand anxiety and learn about applied psychophysiological therapeutic approaches that achieve relatively rapid control over anxiety symptoms, breathing and pain. These approaches are based on a biopsychosocial model of health and involve a combination of cognitive behavior therapy, hypnosis and biofeedback.

Many of the cognitive therapy techniques have been presented in Chapter 3 and this chapter. The hypnosis and biofeedback components of the psychophysiological approach are beyond the scope of this book and require training and certification for clinical application. However, speech-language pathologists should know about the power of these therapies, and strive to learn more about them by affiliating with biofeedback clinicians or psychologists who are certified in these areas of health care, or get training themselves in biofeedback and/or hypnosis as an adjunctive technique for anxiety-related voice and speech disorders. An excellent source of information is the Association for Applied Psychophysiology and Biofeedback (AAPB):

Association for Applied Psychophysiology and Biofeedback
10200 W. 44th Ave.
Suite 304
Wheatridge, CO 80033-2840
http://www.aapb.org

Unfortunately, there is very little crossover between the fields of speech-language pathology and applied psychophysiology. This is particularly regrettable because there is also very promising work by psychophysiologists in the use of EEG (neurotherapy) with attentional deficits (ADD), strokes, and closed head injuries, patient populations that speech clinicians traditionally treat. Interesting work is also being done in pain control with EEG, which has significance for voice specialists, who frequently encounter this problem (odyphonia) with little success.

Recent Advances in Anxiety Management

Speech-language pathologists and others interested in communication apprehension should also be aware of recent advances in psychophysiology pertaining to anxiety reduction, specifically respiratory sinus arrhythmia (RSA) training. They should also follow the rapid advances in bio-vir, the marriage of biofeedback and virtual reality, an innovative therapy to treat anxiety.

Respiratory Sinus Arrhythmia

The recent work on RSA in the field of physiology, mentioned briefly in this chapter and Chapters 3 and 4, has significance for the field of communication disorders. Respiration is regulated to maintain the correct partial pressures of O_2 and CO_2 in the arterial blood, which ensures the transport of these gases to and from tissues. RSA is the variation in heart rate that accompanies breathing and is one of the several identified oscillatory mechanisms in heart rhythm.

According to Smetankin, a Russian physiologist, there has been a tendency to consider the control of the respiratory and cardiovascular systems as if they were independent of each other (personal communication). However, there is increasing evidence that the two systems are very closely linked. The most obvious manifestation of the linkage is the cyclic variations in heart rate during inspiration (heart rate increases) and expiration (heart rate decreases). Synchronization of the two systems is considered the most important element in restoring autonomic homeostasis (sympathetic/parasympathetic balance). According to Porges (1986) RSA is used as an index of parasympathetic tone and is related to self-regulation (Porges, 1995). The numerical value of RSA is known to differ with age and individual function. The higher the RSA, the better the state of homeostasis at any age.

RSA Training For the past several years, the Russians (Smetankin, 1997) have used the small portable biofeedback instrument (a heart tracker) called a cardiosignalizer, mentioned earlier in this chapter, to teach patients to synchronize their breathing and heart rate. Beginning with slow diaphragmatic breathing, the synchrony is reflected in visual and auditory signals on the cardiosignalizer. They report that this biofeedback training (15 days for 20 minutes/day), results in a significant increase of the RSA amplitude, indicating that patients have succeeded in synchronizing their breathing with their heart rate. According to Russian research, this training permanently changes the patients' homeostasis which is reflected in positive changes in muscle tension, brain wave activity (alpha states), body temperature, and skin conductance. Smetankin (personal communication) also reports these physiological changes result in a reduction of negative thoughts and greater self-confidence. The new, habituated breathing pattern is then used in anticipation of and during actual stressful situations.

RSA biofeedback has been used in Russia to treat stuttering and asthma (Kiseleva, Vovk, 1998; Lehrer, Smetankin, & Potapova, 2000; Smetankin, 1999; Smetankin, Bourmistrov, Vovk, & Horwitz, 2000; Smetankin, Vovk, Bourmistrov, Horwitz, & Spiridonov, 1999; Trufakina, 1998; Vovk, 1999) and to reduce autonomic hyperarousal in patients with anxiety (Chernigovshaya, Vaschillo, Rusanovsky, & Kashkarovka, 1990). This technique has not yet been tested in controlled studies, but shows promise as a more rapid and direct route for calming the nervous system. Clinical trials are now being conducted on this and a similar approach with asthma patients at the University of Medicine and Dentistry of New Jersey and the California School of Professional Psychology.

Lehrer, Vaschillo, and Vaschillo (2000) are training persons with asthma to control their anxiety and symptoms with the cardiosignalizer as well as with other heartrate biofeedback instrumentation

(C2 and DSP-12 with special software) that reflects RSA changes in a spectral analysis of heart rhythm. As with RSA training, clients are taught to slow their breathing and to take breaths diaphragmatically, in a relaxed and natural way, so that the abdomen expands when inhaling and contracts when exhaling. The researchers believe systematic alterations in the spectral patterns of the heart that occurs with RSA account for the restoration of homeostatic reflexes, muscle recovery, cardiopulmonary function, and baroreceptor sensitivity. Therefore, they call their work resonant frequency training (RFT), rather than RSA training. They also attribute the modulation of the autonomic activity that occurs to changes in different heart frequencies, resulting in a resonance (greatly increased amplitude of oscillation) at a low frequency as well as to greater baroreflex efficiency.

In summary, RSA and RFT training hold promise for helping people with communication apprehension and other anxiety-related speech and voice disorders. These approaches offer a monitored, direct, and, perhaps, permanent way of reducing hyperarousal. According to Smetankin (personal communication), there is no way to ensure that these ancient breathing techniques used in yoga and meditation techniques result in synchronization of the cardiovascular and respiratory systems necessary for reestablishment of homeostasis unless RSA changes occur. Tracking and measuring the two systems with a cardiosignalizer or other heart tracking instrumentation is the only way to ensure that increases in RSA actually occur (Lehrer, Smetankin, et al., 2000).

Virtual Reality Therapy

Virtual reality[2] was developed in the mid-to-late 1980s, and its potential for the treatment of psychological disorders was noted shortly afterwards (North, North, & Coble, 1996). Virtual reality training (VRT) is a technology that enables a patient to enter computer-generated worlds and interact with various environments through sight, sound, and touch. It can provide a patient with a sense of presence or immersion in a feared situation. In general, VRT is an efficient means of directly treating a variety of phobias.

The VRT 2003® unit includes a head-mounted display with a head-tracking unit and tactile devices to produce visual, auditory, and tactile stimuli. Specific VRT scenes are used for a multitude of situations and

---

[2]an artificial environment experienced through sensory stimulation by a computer and in which a user's actions partially determine what happens in the "virtual" environment

provide a safe and effective environment for research and or services. It has been used effectively for treatment of agoraphobia (scary situations such as elevators, bridges, dark and or empty barn scenes, etc.), acrophobia (fear of heights), and fear of flying. The Speech Improvement Company in Boston has also used it with patients who feared public speaking (communication apprehension) with a virtual auditorium and audience, accompanied by visual and audio responses.

The virtual reality system gives speakers the experience of being in front of a virtual auditorium, which gradually fills with virtual people. Simulation of a room and crowd noises, including laughter, commentary, and applause is created and experienced as part of the treatment session.

The symptoms experienced by a speaker during such a session mirror those that most speakers feel during a presentation in front of a large group (e.g., increased heart rate, dry mouth, sweaty palms, difficulty breathing, etc.). A specially trained coach monitors and guides the session, introducing appropriate speaking techniques. Periodic subjective reports are elicited to closely monitor progress, behavior, and reactions. Five to eight hour-long sessions are conducted during the treatment. Individual progress dictates the length and intensity of each session (North, North, and Coble, 1998).

VRT is still being refined and presently is expensive ($10,000 for a system). However, researchers are working on developing inexpensive, flexible, and reliable systems, while increasing the functionality and usefulness of the system. This author (B. H.) has experienced the virtual reality system for fear of flying at the School of Professional Psychology in San Diego, CA, and can attest to its ability to realistically simulate actual flying conditions (landing, taking off, turbulence, etc.). This therapy has exciting prospects for reducing fears in many situations, especially performance and other social and speaking fears.

Chapter Summary

Communication apprehension, a transient somatized reaction to specific social fears, can be effectively managed in a small group that addresses its psychphysiological etiology as well as cognitive, physiological and behavioral strategies to reduce the fear. The program for business and professional people that was presented can be adapted for use with other populations that suffer performance anxiety as well as with some communication disorders, especially dysfluency and selected voice disorders. The most recent treatment modalities for anxiety reduction including RSA/RFT training and virtual reality which were explained also hold promise for future treatment of performance anxiety.

References

Bless, D., Swift, E., Swift, W., Pasic, T., & Sandage, M. (1999, November). *A new look at assessment and treatment of paradoxical vocal cord dysfunction (PVCD)*. Workshop presented at the annual meeting of the American Speech and Hearing Association, San Francisco.

Bourne, E. (1995). *The anxiety and phobia workbook*. Oakland, CA: Harbinger Press.

Cannon, W. B. (1953). *Bodily changes in pain, hunger, fear and rage*. Boston: C. T. Branford.

Carson, R. D. (1983). *Taming your gremlin: A guide to enjoying yourself*. New York: Harper & Row.

Chernigovshaya, N., Vaschillo, E. G., Rusanovsky, B. B., & Kashkarovka, O. E. (1990). Instrumental autotraining of mechanisms for cardiovascular function regulation in treatment of neurotics (Russian). *The SS Korsakovi Journal of Neuropathology and Psychiatry, 90*, 24–28.

Crown, D. P. & Marlowe, D. (1960). A new scale of social desirability independent of psychopathology. *Journal of Consulting Psychology, 24*, 349–354.

Davids, K. L., Smith, S., & Montgomery, D. D. (1996). Two case studies using EMG biofeedback treatment for laryngeal spasms and psychogenic hyperfunctinal voice disorder (abstract). *Journal of Biofeedback and Self-Regulation, 21*, 353.

Everly, G. S., Jr. & Rosenfeld, R. (1981). *The nature and treatment of the stress response: A practical guide for clinicians*. New York: Plenum.

Eysenck, H. J. & Eysenck, B. J. (1976). *Eysenck Personality Questionnaire-R*. San Diego: Edits/Educational and Industrial Testing Service.

Fried, R. (1990). *The breath connection: How to reduce psychosomatic and stress-related disorders with easy-to-do breathing exercises*. New York: Insight Books.

Girdano, D. & Everly, G. (1979). *Controlling stress and tension: A holistic approach*. Englewood Cliffs, NJ: Prentice-Hall.

Greene, C. (1998). *Audition success*. New York: Pro Mind Music.

Hickerson, J. C. (1997). *A biofeedback/cognitive-behavioral treatment model for women with public speaking anxiety*. Unpublished doctoral dissertation, University of Texas, Arlington.

Hickerson, J. & Shannon, C. (1998). *Scared speechless: Treating public speaking anxiety utilizing biofeedback*. Workshop presented at the Association of Applied Psychophysiology and Biofeedback meeting, Orlando, FL.

Jacobson, E. (1974). *Progressive relaxation*. Chicago: The University of Chicago Press, Midway Reprint.

Kiseleva, M. N. & Vovk, O. N. (1998). On treatment of adult stammerers by the biofeedback method. In M. B. Shtark & R. Kall (Eds.), *Biofeedback—3* (pp. 87–96). Novosibirsk: Institute of Medical and Biological Cybernetics, Siberian Department of Russian Academy of Medical Science.

Lehrer, P., Smetankin, A., & Potapova, T. (2000). Respiratory sinus arrhythmia biofeedback for asthma: A report of 20 unmedicated pediatric cases using the Smetankin Method. *Applied Psychophysiology and Biofeedback, 25,* 193–200.

Lehrer, P., Vaschillo, E., & Vaschillo, B. (2000). Resonant frequency biofeedback training to increase cardiac variability: Rationale and manual for training. *Applied Psychophysiology and Biofeedback, 25,* 177–191.

Levelt, W. J. M. (1989). *Speaking: From intention to articulation.* Cambridge: MIT Press.

McCroskey, J. C. (2001). *An introduction to rhetorical communication* (8th ed.). Needham Heights, MA: Allyn & Bacon.

McCroskey, J. C. & Richmond, V. (1979). The impact of communication apprehension on individuals in organizations. *Communication Quarterly, 27,* 55–61.

McCroskey, J. C. & Richmond, V. (1980). The quiet ones: Communication apprehension and shyness. In W. Arnold (Ed.), *Components in speech communication* (pp. 19–21). Dubuque, IA: Gorsuch Scarisbrick Publishers.

North, M. M., North, S. M., & Coble, J. R. (1996). *Virtual reality therapy: An innovative paradigm.* Colorado Springs, CO: IPI Press.

North, M. M., North, S. M., & Coble, J. R. (1998). Virtual reality therapy: An effective treatment for fear of public speaking. *International Journal of Vitural Reality, 3 (2),* p. 2–6.

Peters, H. F. M. (1998, August). *Speech motor research in stuttering: Some reflections.* Paper presented at the seminar, Research and Treatment in Stuttering at the 24th Congress of the International Association of Logopedics and Phoniatrics (IALP), Amsterdam, NL.

Porges, S. W. (1986). Respiratory sinus arrhythmia: Physiological basis, quantitative methods and clinical implications. In P. Grossman, K. Janssen, & D. Vaitl (Eds.), *Cardiorespiratory and cardiosomatic psychophysiology* (pp. 101–115). New York: Plenum Press.

Porges, S. W. (1995). Orienting in a defensive world: Mamallian modifications of our evolutionary heritage. A polyvagal theory. *Psychophysiology, 32,* 301–318.

Schneier, F. & Welkowitz, L. (1996). *The hidden face of shyness.* New York: Avon Books.

Sifneos, P. M. (1972). *Short-term psychotherapy and emotional crisis.* Cambridge, MA: Harvard University Press.

Sime, W. & Healey, E. C. (1993). An interdisciplinary approach to the treatment of a hyperfunctional voice disorder. *Biofeedback and Self-Regulation, 18,* 1–7.

Smetankin, A. (1997, Summer). Biofeedback developments in Russia: Progress in the biofeedback treatment of childhood asthma. *Biofeedback News Magazine, 25,* 8–11, 17.

Smetankin, A. (1999). The use of RSA biofeedback in speech formation for speech pathology and healthy people. *Biologicheskaya Obratnaya Svyaz, No. 2,* 3–14.

Smetankin, A., Bourmistrov, A., Vovk, O., & Horwitz, B. (2000). *New method of speech correction using RSA biofeedback.* Presentatation at a meeting of the International Fluency Association, Nyborg, Denmark.

Smetankin, A., Vovk, O., Bourmistrov, A., Horwitz, B., & Spiridonov, E. (1999). Comparative evaluation of breathing patterns and heart rate changes in speech/voice/language specialists from Russia and the USA during shaping diaphragmatic-relaxation breating by the RSA-biofeedback method. *Biologicheskaya Obratnaya Svyaz, No. 2,* 22–33.

Stroebel, C. F. (1982). *QR: The quieting reflex.* New York: Putnam.

Swift, W. J. (1999, November). *Psychiatric aspects of paradoxical vocal cord dysfunction (PVCD).* Workshop presented at the annual meeting of the American Speech and Hearing Association, San Francisco.

Tellegen, A. & Atkinson, G. (1974). Openness to absorbing and self-altering experiences ("absorption"): A trait related to hypnotic susceptibility. *Journal of Abnormal Psychology, 83,* 268–277.

Trufakina, L. V. (1998). On the use of biofeedback in logopedia for speech correction among preschool children suffering from stammer. In M. B. Shtark & R. Kall (Eds.), *Biofeedback—3* (pp. 96–101). Novosibirsk: Institute of Medical and Biological Cybernetics, Siberian Department of Russian Academy of Medical Science.

Vovk, O. (1999). On biofeedback treatment of adult stutterers. *Biologicheskaya Obratnaya Svyaz, No. 2,* 15–21.

Wickramasekera, I. (1988). *Clinical behavioral medicine: Some concepts and procedures.* New York: Plenum Press.

Wickramasekera, I. (1998). Secrets kept from the mind but not the body or behavior: The unsolved problems of identifying and treating somatization and psychophysiological disease. *Advances in Mind-Body Medicine, 14,* 81–132.

Wickramasekera, I. (1999). How does biofeedback reduce clinical symptoms and do memories and beliefs have biological consequences? Toward a model of mind-body healing. *Journal of Applied Psychophysiology and Biofeedback, 24,* 91–105.

Zocco, L. (1984). *The development of a self-report inventory to assess dysfunctional cognitions in phobics.* Unpublished doctoral dissertation, Virginia Consortium for Professional Psychology, Virginia Beach, VA.

Suggested Readings

*Required reading

*Carson, R. (1983). *Taming your gremlin: A guide to enjoying yourself.* New York: Harper Perennial.

Criswell-Hanna, E. (1995). *Biofeedback and somatics: Toward personal evolution.* Novato, CA: Freeperson Press.

Everly, G. S., Jr. & Girdano, D. A. (1980). *The stress mess solution.* Bowie, MD: R. J. Brady Co.

Fried, R. (1999). *Breathe well, be well: A program to relieve stress, anxiety, asthma, hypertension, migraine, and other disorders for better health.* New York: John Wiley & Sons.

*Gronbeck, B. E., Ehninger, D., & Monroe, A. H. (1988). *Principles of speech communication.* Glenview, IL: Scott, Foresman.

*Handly, R. (1985). *Anxiety and panic attacks: Their cause and cure.* New York: Rawson Associates.

Linden, W. (1990). *Autogenic training: A clinical guide.* New York: The Guilford Press.

McKay, M., Davis, M., & Fanning, P. (1997). *Thoughts and feelings: Taking control of your moods and your life.* Oakland, CA: New Harbinger Publications, Inc.

Sapolsky, R. (1998). *Why zebras don't get ulcers: An updated guide to stress, stress-related diseases, and coping.* New York: W. H. Freeman and Co.

Schneier, F. & Welkowitz, L. (1996). *The hidden face of shyness.* New York: Avon Books.

Sedlack, K. (1989). *Sedlack technique: Finding the calm within you.* New York: McGraw Hill.

Appendix 5-1

SPEAKING WITHOUT FEAR
Simply Noticing

Name: Date:

As you spoke:
   What were you thinking?

   What were you feeling?

Rate your level of fear from 1 (low) to 10 (high)_____

If you can, draw your fear (stick figures or diagrams will do).

Dr. Betty Horwitz, NYU, SCPS 2001

Appendix 5-2

SPEAKING WITHOUT FEAR
Identifying Information

Name: Date:

Address:

Phone Home: Office: E-Mail:

Place of Birth: Years in U.S.A.:

Educational background:

Previous speech courses:

Vocation:

Speaking responsibilities on the job:

Reason for taking the course:

Pertinent medical problems:

Medications:

Counseling, psychotherapy:

To what do you attribute your fear of speaking?

Comments and questions:

Dr. Betty Horwitz, NYU, SCPS 2001

Appendix 5-3

What If Exercise

Name: Date:

Instructions: Complete question #1 (If I?) with a speaking situation you would ordinarily avoid. After "Then," record what you think would happen if you actually took the risk. Continue to record situations and what you think the consequences would be for each previous statement. Note how realistic your feelings and fears are.

Example:
If I: raised my hand
Then: I would be called on

If: I am called on
Then: I would have to respond

and so on... .

1. If I?_____

   Then:_____

2. If (that happens)_____

   Then:_____

3. If (that happens)_____

   Then:_____

4. If (that happens)_____

   Then:_____

5. If (that happens)_____

   Then_____

6. If (that happens)_____

   Then_____

Dr. Betty Horwitz, NYU, SCPS 2001

Appendix 5-4

Psychophysiological Diary

Name: Date:

Column One: Describe the events that appear to trigger your fearful reaction to speaking.
Column Two: Identify your automatic, negative thoughts about speaking in each situation.
Column Three: Record any physical changes, symptoms, or reactions following each event.

1 **Event** **Reactions** (Person or event that upset you when speaking)	2 **Cognitions** (Thoughts, worries, and interpretations of that event)	3 **Physical** **Reactions** (Physical changes, symptoms, and signs that accompanied your thoughts)

Action: Mark with an asterisk (*) any cognition that you want to "catch," stop, and modify. Remember the typical distortions in thinking that cause dysfunctional responses to stress.

Identify Distortions: 1. All or nothing thinking 2. Overgeneralizations 3. Mental filters 4. Discounting the positives 5. Mind reading 6. Fortune telling 7. Magnification of minimization 8. Emotional reasoning 9. Should statements 10. Labeling 11. Personalization and blame

Note: Copyright by Dr. Donald Moss, Ph.D., 1992, Psychological Services Center. Adapted with Permission.

Appendix 5-5

Designing A Hierarchy of Speaking Fears

Name: Date:

FEAR HIERARCHY

This hierarchy is like a ladder that one climbs from the bottom up. Approaching things one step at a time makes progress possible. Therefore, begin at the bottom by first writing the situations and people triggering even the slightest anxiety or fear about social situations and/or speaking. As you work upward, list situations and people provoking more anxiety, from the least to the most, which will be at the top.

Most Anxiety Provoking

Least Anxiety Provoking

On your own, begin speaking and dealing socially in these situations and with these people, starting with the least fearful event. You might begin by first asking a question or making a comment. Work up to a point where you can gradually increase your participation and become a major contributor, even volunteering to conduct meetings or to give presentations where appropriate. Overcoming the fear of speaking is a gradual process that must begin now. Take responsibility for your own progress and keep careful records of your participation noting what occurred and how you felt.

Dr. Betty Horwitz, NYU, SCPS 2001

CHAPTER

6

Epilogue

What Is Known

Communication apprehension is a universal, common problem with a multiplicity of causes and degrees of severity. At last, something of its physiological origin is now known—namely that it is a somatized reaction to a specific class of social stressors which includes speaking in public. The physiological symptoms of communication apprehension result from withdrawal of the vagal tone by the "smart vagus," according to the polyvagal theory of the autonomic nervous system (See Gevirtz, Chapter 4), which innervates the somatic musculature of the palate, larynx, pharynx, and esophagus. It is also known that anxiety results in rapid and shallow breathing that leads to a change in the acid-base balance of the body (to more alkaline), which interferes with the release of oxygen from hemoglobin and ultimately hampers cortical activity. These physiological actions result in a reduction of cortical blood flow, vasoconstriction, activation of the cardiovascular system, increase in muscle tone, and even gastrointestinal disruption. When that physiological response is prolonged, it leads to reduced clarity thinking and other well-known symptoms of communication apprehension.

Even more is known about the psychological triggers and profound social and professional repercussions of communication apprehension, documented throughout this volume. Also understood is how to deal with the problem in a cost-effective way, using a top-down approach with cognitive/behavioral, affective, and physiological targets and communication skills training.

What Needs to be Known

The Topdown approach used in the class Speaking Without Fear was indeed effective for most participants in the class. However, some individuals did not improve as dramatically as others for a variety of reasons. It is apparent that there is a clear need to differentiate among clients to develop clearer treatment protocols for individual and group treatment. This can be accomplished by assessment procedures that include psychological and physiological profiles of individuals pre- and post-therapy. This requires the use of some biofeedback equipment, at minimum an EMG instrument that measures the level of muscle tension. In addition, routine temperature and GSR measures, as well as several questionnaires about types and severity of communication apprehension and progress would be useful.

Research studies of groups formed on the bases of psychological profiles, with controls, should be conducted to determine the effectiveness of various therapeutic strategies including top-down and bottom-up approaches (See Wickramasekera). Systematic records of changes in thought and fear ratings should be maintained. There is also a need for follow-up studies to determine maintenance of treatment progress for all groups.

Finally, there is an exciting opportunity to study and compare the new approaches to anxiety reduction, such as RSA, or RFT training, to determine if this therapy can hasten and maintain homeostasis and positive thinking, as the Russian reports claim. The efficacy of virtual reality training with communication apprehension is also a promising approach for the future that should be investigated.

What Needs to be Done

This is a time of great opportunity for speech-language pathologists interested in broadening their scope of knowledge and practice. Programs for communication apprehension should be implemented because the population in need is enormous at all ages and levels of education. They should be introduced into the upper primary grades to identify and prevent escalation of the problem later in life. Perhaps, as with phonological awareness and language stimulation programs, speech-language pathologists should be integrating speaking-anxiety-reduction and self-regulation programs into elementary school curricula, encouraging more oral communication in the classes, and conducting workshops for teachers on the problem of social phobia.

In addition, because communication apprehension is so prevalent, university speech-language clinics might consider integrating normally fluent anxious speakers and dysfluent speakers into the same group program or establish separate programs for students suffering this hidden disability.

Finally, all music and drama departments and special schools for the performing arts should set up substantive programs for performance anxiety. The basic problems for talented, aspiring performers do not differ substantially from those of other people, although they certainly are subject to special pressures in their professional fields. Such performance anxiety programs should be adapted to meet the needs and types of talents (singers versus instrumentalists), but should always include information on the origins and physiology of anxiety, as well as all the therapeutic means to overcome communication apprehension presented in this book, including the use of selected biofeedback instrumentation. Aspiring and working performers should be helped to face the rigors of intense competition and to recognize and control the symptoms of anxiety that interfere with their performance before they become discouraged or self-sabotage their careers. Some exciting investigations on performance anxiety with musicians have been conducted with good information and implications for treatment (Zinn, 2000; Sataloff, 1999; McEwen, 1998; Zinn, McCaine, and Zinn 2000; Fredrickson and Gunnarsson, 1992).

Reflections

The recent work in the neural sciences on fear is voluminous and has shed light on the mind-body connection and the treatment of anxiety-related disorders including performance anxiety. The next sections recap some of the basic tenets underlying the origin and management of communication apprehension presented in this book.

- Modern methods of brain function and information on brain chemistry make it increasingly apparent that psychology (behavior) is grounded in biology.

- There is nothing in an organism's behavior that is purely physical or organic. Behavior, thoughts, emotions, and socialization are mirrored in physiological processes, which are a window to the brain.

- Survival today is no longer a matter of warding off dangerous predators, but depends on social relationships and events—socialization with other people, who often represent a threat or challenge, depending on how an individual perceives the people and the social context.

- Human beings are group animals who depend on each other for safety. Therefore, the social evaluative aspect of living is an integral part of our being to which the ANS and the endocrine system respond. Hence, our need for approval and support.
- Performing in front of others can be perceived as a dangerous event, in part because some people correlate being looked at with being threatened.
- The behavior and values of human beings are the result of inborn tendencies and learning, as well as acquired through observation and indoctrination by members of their cultural group.
- Beliefs, expectations, and attitudes play critical roles in the way the world is viewed and how individuals perform or behave.
- Anxiety is a natural adaptive response to fear, real or perceived, whose primary purpose is to alert and protect an individual, increasing his or her chance of survival.
- The stress response is the brain's way of protecting the organism.
- The brain confronts novelty by calling on the stress response, thereby increasing an individual's readiness to deal with a threat. Reducing novelty through education and awareness can reduce stress.
- Emotions stem from hormones that are released into the blood-stream and are responsible for many stress symptoms, often without a person's awareness of their existence or cause.
- Warm-blooded mammals, unlike cold-blooded animals, such as reptiles, are capable of physiological self-regulation.
- Respiration is a key to reducing arousal of the ANS and the endocrine system. It reflects and affects states of consciousness and is fundamental to teaching and achieving relaxation.

Professional Directions

Individually and organizationally, speech language pathologists can responsibly serve a wider client base by:

- Understanding the origins and management of communication apprehension and recognizing it as a serious communication disorder that SLPs should treat.
- Considering the early identification and prevention of communication apprehension a part of professional responsibility
- Having ASHA or special interest groups consider communication apprehension within the scope of practice and offering training on the topic.

- Incorporating assessment and therapy procedures for social anxiety into speech assessment and treatment protocols when necessary, especially with voice and fluency disorders.
- Growing beyond the traditional medical model of disorders and recognizing the power and significance of the mind-body connection, the ancient and modern approach to health and effective performance.
- Considering the person, the whole person, not just a disorder when treating someone with a speech or voice problem.
- Establishing liaisons with applied psychophysiological clinics or offering graduate course work in psychophysiology and biofeedback so that SLP students can learn about behavioral medicine and its implications for the field of speech and voice pathology.

References

Fredrickson, M. & Gunnarsson, G. (1992). Psychobiology of stage fright. The effect of public performance on neuroendocrine, cardiovascular and subjective reactions. *Biological Psychology, 33,* 51–61.

McEwen, B. (1998). Protective and damaging effects of stress mediators. *New England Journal of Medicine, 338,* 171–179.

Sataloff, R. T., Rosen, D. C., & Levy S. (1999). A comprehensive approach. *Medical Problems of Performing Artists, 14,* 122–126.

Zinn, M., McCaine, C., & Zinn, M. (2000). Musical performance anxiety and the high risk model of threat perception. *Medical Problems of Performing Artists, 15,* 65–71.

Zinn, M. (2000). Professional music teachers and the high risk model of threat perception: Some data and predictions. *Applied Psychophysiology and Biofeedback, 25,* 258.

INDEX

Note: *Italicized page numbers refer to tables and figures.*